T0167569

CRYSTAL
PRESCRIPTIONS

Volume 3

Crystal solutions to electromagnetic
pollution and geopathic stress
An A-Z guide

Volumes in this series

CRYSTAL
PRESCRIPTIONS

Volume 3

Crystal solutions to electromagnetic
pollution and geopathic stress
An A-Z guide

Judy Hall

Author of the best-selling

The Crystal Bible series

BOOKS

Winchester, UK
Washington, USA

JOHN HUNT PUBLISHING

First published by O-Books, 2014
O-Books is an imprint of John Hunt Publishing Ltd., 3 East St., Alresford,
Hampshire SO24 9EE, UK
office@jhpbooks.com
www.johnhuntpublishing.com
www.o-books.com

For distributor details and how to order please visit the 'Ordering' section on
our website.

ISBN: 978 1 78279 791 3
978 1 78279 790 6 (ebook)

A CIP catalogue record for this book is available from the British Library.

Design: Stuart Davies

UK: Printed and bound by CPI Group (UK) Ltd, Croydon, CR0 4YY
Printed in North America by CPI GPS partners

We operate a distinctive and ethical publishing philosophy
in all areas of our business, from our global network of
authors to production and worldwide distribution.

CONTENTS

This third A–Z directory by the author of *The Crystal Bibles* explores the effects of electromagnetic field (EMF) pollution and geopathic stress (GS) on health and well-being, and the dis-eases and healing crystals associated with them. Including 20 crystal portraits, the directory assists in identifying the right crystal for your needs whether it is for personal energetic support and healing for EMF and GS effects, or environmental protection against electromagnetic and geopathic stress. With practical applications, the directory also includes essential information on keeping your crystals working for you.

Disclaimer

The information given in this directory is in no way intended to be a substitute for treatment by a medical practitioner. Further assistance can also be sought from a suitably qualified crystal healer or anti-geopathic stress practitioner. Healing can be defined as bringing the body, emotions, mind and spirit back into balance. It does not imply a cure.

Acknowledgements

My particular thanks go to New Zealand Geomancer Nicky Crocker for so generously sharing her research findings with me and allowing me to publish them here, and to Professor Denis Henshaw who graciously gave permission to quote from his research. Thanks are also due to the many lecturers, practitioners and interested parties with whom I have discussed the effects of geopathic stress and electromagnetic hypersensitivity over the past thirty-five or so years. And to those who make their findings accessible through the World Wide Web, all power to you. Workshop participants and clients in many countries have helped me to explore the properties of crystals, blessings to you all.

Introduction:

Living in an energetically polluted world

A hundred years from now, we will look back at pylons as relics of the mid-20th century. It probably won't happen in five or ten years, but eventually a new generation will come along, change things, and wonder why we did nothing.
– Professor Denis Henshaw, Bristol University[1]

Everything on Earth resonates at a vibrational frequency. Frequency basically means the rate at which the molecules, or atoms, of matter rotate around one another, creating an energetic wave or vibration. The human vibrational field operates in harmony with all other beings – animals, plants, minerals and the planet itself – and has to be maintained at a specific level to ensure optimal health and well-being. This synergistic bioenergy, including our auric and physiological structure, can be disturbed by disorganised and disharmonious frequencies. Modern technologies and communication devices rely on electromagnetic waves in order to carry out their function. The frequencies these generate can affect human vibrations, leading to the disturbance of our inner biological clock, compromised immunity and a drop in overall well-being.

I live in a house protected by more than a few crystals. Essential as there is an electricity substation nearby. Since attending the Baden Baden Medicine Fair in the 1990s, where electromagnetic fields (EMFs) and geopathic stress (GS) as a cause of dis-ease were regularly discussed, and speaking to researchers, healers and doctors working at the cutting edge of energy medicine, I am well aware that EMFs can have a seriously detrimental effect on health, as may GS. The evidence is increasing year on year. We'll be taking a look at it a little later.

My computer, which is surrounded by crystals, runs a programme to counteract its EMF effects and put out healing for myself and the surrounding area. The need for EMF protection was apparent when I had my very first computer. I felt that it drew all the energy from me, leading to rapid exhaustion. But, also, it kept crashing. Clearly something was wrong. The computer engineer also happened to be a martial arts instructor and had a good understanding of how subtle energy works. Having first ascertained that there were no ghosts in the property, he gave his considered opinion: "psychics and computers don't mix." It would appear that my energy was interfering with the computer in the same way that it was interfering with mine; the two were incompatible. Agreed. But unfortunately writers and modern-day publishers have to communicate via the Internet, and I often write on a computer for many hours a day. Fortunately for me, Victor Sims was at the time designing the amazing Computer Clear program which I've used ever since.[2] It utilises the energetic signature of a number of crystals as well as flower essences and homeopathic remedies to strengthen your body's natural resistance to EMF radiation. As Victor puts it, "[the] patterns have been specially selected during the many years of research. Every imbalance in the body has a complementary energetic pattern that will bring it back to optimum health; the body's consciousness is autonomous and responds by sympathetic resonance to accept the patterns that it needs from Computer Clear. Each pattern that the body resonates with 'kick starts' a particular part of the body's healing system allowing it to return to homeostasis." I couldn't work without it, and the same applies to my crystals, which perform a similar task in a similar way.

I've found plane travel particularly taxing, especially long-distance flights – not only does the pressurisation and the poor quality of oxygen affect me but also the fact that a plane acts like an electrosmog generator that has nowhere to discharge itself, all the worse now for the proliferation of cell phones and computers on board. And then there is the horror of full body scanners and X-ray overload. Fortunately wearing Shungite and Preseli Bluestone negates the effect and reconnects me to Earth when I land. But it is not only man-made electromagnetic smog that may cause problems. The ground under our feet carries its own geopathic energy, which may be distorted or stressed. Hence the term geopathic stress (GS) which translates as 'suffering earth'.

Living on a magnetic Earth

So why do we need protecting from what may be very weak electromagnetic fields but which on occasion may be distorted to as high as 250 Hz? Well, the correct functioning of our biological rhythms, cell metabolism, physiological state and mental well-being depends on communication between the electrical system of our brain, body and endocrine system, and the weak electromagnetic and magnetic fields generated by the planet. And, our bodies are full of magnetisable materials such as the iron in our blood. Life on Earth evolved against the natural electromagnetic field of the planet and so human beings are accustomed to living within its background oscillation at a frequency of around 7.83 Hz and can adapt to the slight fluctuations in the field created by electrical storms, magnetic irregularities and solar activity. However, larger fluctuations in electromagnetic and geopathic energy may be detrimental to the health of human beings. As Rolf Gordon of Dulwich Health, a pioneering researcher of the effects of GS, puts it, "GS does not cause an illness, but lowers your immune system, so you have less chance of fighting any illness. GS also prevents your body properly absorbing vitamins, minerals, trace elements etc. from your food (and supplements), often making you allergic to food, drinks and environmental pollution."[3] How we know that they are damaging is revealed through the ever-increasing flow of scientific evidence from around the world as well as from anecdotal evidence spread over the last century (see pages 23, 28, and 131 and Research Findings Report at the end of the book), but GS is nothing new. It was identified several thousand years ago by Chinese geomancers who created a system of Feng Shui to harmonise it.

Geopathic stress

Earth and physiological stress created by subtle emanations and vibrational conflicts or disturbances from underground water, power lines, natural landscape features, negative earth energy and other subterranean events.

Living in smog

In our modern-day world geopathic stress and subtle energy pathogens surround us virtually everywhere. We are enveloped in constant man-made electromagnetic smog, an intrusive and detectable electromagnetic field given off by power lines, Wi-Fi and electrical equipment that has an adverse effect on sensitive people as it raises the background oscillation frequency way beyond what the human body is adapted to deal with. Since the discovery of electricity we have been increasingly exposed to a wide range of powerful, artificially generated, electromagnetic radiation that adversely affects the Earth's energy field and the human body. Nor are we adapted to mobile phone signals and high frequency transmissions. As a result, this sudden onslaught has been accompanied by an exponential rise in the 'diseases of civilisation', cancer, diabetes, heart attacks, chronic fatigue syndrome, irritable bowel, Parkinson's and the like, all of which are now being shown to be consequences of electromagnetic sensitivity and geopathic stress.[4]

Electromagnetic smog

A subtle but detectable electromagnetic field given off by power lines and electrical equipment that has an adverse effect on sensitive people.

Planetary and physiological stress is created by energetic disturbance from underground water, power lines and ley lines, and human activity such as mining or construction. You may ask why these energetic intrusions matter. Well, every cell in our body has its own electrical system and the human body, as with all living things including crystals, is surrounded and interpenetrated by a subtle, organised electromagnetic energy field known as the aura or biomagnetic sheath. Our bioenergy interacts with the subtle energy fields that surround it. These fields must be in harmony to maintain well-being; distortions create dis-ease. Researchers have recently discovered important – and delicate – communication mechanisms within the cellular structure itself that can be damaged by EMF frequencies (see page 40). In conventional medicine there has been a general lack of awareness and understanding of the impact electromagnetic fields and geopathic stress can have upon health and well-being, but this is being rectified as more doctors and scientists become aware and in-depth research takes place.

I've spent considerable time researching GS, ley lines and the siting of ancient sacred sites – and their connection with crystals. As T. Saunders has pointed out:

> our ancestors were acutely aware that certain locations were perceived to have a positive energy field which was beneficial to health and vitality. Over time, these areas are now referred to as sacred sites for spiritual ceremony and as healing centres. In contrast, there are other geographical locations that may have a negative effect upon health and these are known as geopathic stress zones.[5]

> ### Sick building syndrome
> A condition caused by a building with air pollution or inadequate ventilation, excess static electricity, electromagnetic smog, geopathic stress and the like. Symptoms include lack of concentration, headache, chest and skin problems, nausea, excessive fatigue, dizziness.

So, it is clear to me that both GS and EMFs may adversely affect our health – although bioenergy tools can also facilitate healing. I have been forced to find tools that protect me and my energy field both at home and when I am travelling. Crystals are the perfect energetic tool for me as they can be for you. They support a balanced and healthy bioenergy field and overcome subtle negative electromagnetic effects by superimposing harmonising bio-resonance patterns upon the body's electromagnetic field, returning it to homeostasis.

Getting grounded
One of the best tools for handling EMF and GS sensitivity is to get yourself grounded, in contact with the planet and completely earthed with your lower chakras fully functioning. So many people who suffer from excessive sensitivity have only a toehold in incarnation, barely tolerating being in a physical body and always reaching 'out there' for the answer. So, make contact with

the Earth, make a friend of your body, become comfortable in incarnation and the detrimental effects will lessen significantly. How do you do this? Use your crystals!

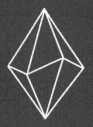

Part I

Environmental sensitivity
and its effects

We have noticed that many people who live close to high voltage power lines suffer sleep disorders and depressive symptoms, an observation which has been seen in a number of professional studies. This could be explained by the fact that magnetic fields such as those found near power lines disrupt the nocturnal production of the important hormone melatonin in the pineal gland... researchers are looking at a number of ways in which both electric and magnetic fields may adversely affect health.
– Professor Denis Henshaw

It's not just human beings that suffer from energetic disruption. Our planet does too. In the same way that the physical body has a measurable bioenergetic sheath around it, linked through the chakras, the Earth has a subtle energy grid surrounding it. This grid is created from and interpenetrated by a complex meridian matrix: intersecting energy lines, some geomagnetic, others electromagnetic, some telluric, others cosmic, that form a global grid through which powerful currents flow. These energies could be called the Earth's Qi or life force. They are like the blood, lymph and chemical messengers of the human physical body, cleansing and revitalising all its organs and stimulating motion. The health and well-being of the Earth and all who reside in or on her body – the planet – depend on the healthy functioning of these fields. These fields may not be in harmony, particularly where they intersect or interact with significant landscape features or man-made structures such as electricity pylons, buildings or quarries. If the grid is broken, disrupted or blocked in any way, especially by GS or the intrusive activities of humankind, the environment suffers. Anyone sensitive who is living there will feel out of sorts, disconnected and unnourished. Their body will also suffer. The effect is found not only in the ground, it can radiate many feet into the air so someone living or working at the top of a thirty-three storey building would feel the effect as much, or perhaps even more, than someone on the ground floor. Suitably placed crystals can harmonise, deflect or transmute the resulting GS, bringing conflicting energy currents back into equilibrium. As we will see, the crystals can be placed at the actual intersection of the lines or alongside fault lines, or on a map as the fields entrain no matter where in the world you may be. In the same way, EMFs that adversely affect the physical body can be counteracted by beneficial crystal fields.

Electromagnetic Fields

Substations may be an issue. It is because they are surrounded by electromagnetic fields that the equipment and cables they contain produce that they have to be treated with caution. Measured electromagnetic fields such as those produced by substations have been associated with health effects such as cancer, depression, dementia, infertility, miscarriage, heart problems, etc.
– Professor Denis Henshaw

Electromagnetic fields are present everywhere in the environment, but are invisible to the human eye. Natural electric fields can build up through electrical charges associated with thunderstorms and certain geomagnetic anomalies but most detrimental electromagnetic fields are man-made. An electromagnetic field (EMF) is produced by electrically charged objects. An electrofield is created by differences in voltage, the higher the voltage, the stronger the field and the further its effect radiates. A field is defined as the area in which the radiation can have a measurable effect on an object or a body. An electromagnetic field extends upwards, downwards and outwards, and interacts with whatever comes into contact with it. Fields can be measured around leads and cables as well as the electrical goods themselves, a phone or a generating station. Electrical fields may still be measurable when an appliance is switched off but is plugged into the mains. Low frequency electromagnetic fields are present when power flows out of a socket when a computer or television is on standby, for instance. Higher frequency waves transmit information such as television signals, radio waves, or mobile phone signals. Magnetic fields are created by a flowing electrofield and are not present once the current ceases.

Common everyday sources of EMFs include:

- Power lines
- Electricity generating stations
- Wi-Fi
- Smart meters
- Electrical wiring
- Microwave ovens
- Computers
- Cordless or cell phones and towers
- Fluorescent and other lighting
- CCTV cameras

Research findings

Professor Denis Henshaw, former head of the Human Radiation Effects Group at Bristol University, has been examining the role played by electric and magnetic fields associated with the electricity supply for many years. His research concerns the way in which magnetic fields interact with the human body and the effects of corona ions emitted from high voltage power lines. He says that: "these lines produce an electrical field large enough to ionise the air around it – in other words, to strip electrons from atoms. The effect is like nudging a line of dominoes... The result is a line of charged, highly reactive particles streaming away from the power cable." He has measured streams as far away as several kilometres from a line. "Such ions transfer their electric charge to particles of air pollution, making these particles more likely to be trapped in the lung on inhalation."[6]

Professor Henshaw goes on to suggest that the adverse health effects associated with electrohypersensitivity and magnetic exposure could all potentially be explained by circadian rhythm disruption. In 1980 it was found that EMFs affected the activity of the pineal gland and researchers have recently found piezoelectric Calcite crystals in the pineal gland that can be adversely affected by EMFs (see Research Findings Reports). Henshaw points out that "during the past fifteen years scientists have discovered just what an important function [the pineal] gland seems to play. It produces a number of very active chemical substances, including important neuro-hormones. Some affect the actions of most of the other glands in the body, including the pituitary." He explains that: "a main function of the pineal gland is the synthesis of the neurohormone melatonin from the neurochemical serotonin... Melatonin is a broad-spectrum, ubiquitously-acting antioxidant and anti-cancer agent, which also reduces growth of human myeloid leukaemia cells and whose disruption by light-at-night is associated with increased cancer risk." If melatonin production is disrupted, the body cannot maintain good health. Another area of concern for him is that magnetic fields induce electrical currents in the brain that create an electrical imbalance.

Professor Henshaw's comprehensive website, whilst no longer regularly updated, also examines the effect of mobile (cell) phones and other sources of EMF disruption and is one of the best places I have found to connect with academic research from around the world. (See also the Draper Report in the Appendix.)

Geopathic Stress: 'The Abode of the Earth Demons'

The term 'geopathic stress' is used to describe negative energies, also known as 'Noxious Earth Energy', which emanate from the earth and cause discomfort and ill health to those living above. Earth energies can be bad, good or neutral. The surface of the earth is woven with a pattern of etheric threads identical in energy and importance to the acupuncture meridians of the human body. But if you are sleeping on one of these 'crossings' or if they are where you spend a lot of time i.e. at your desk or workplace, they could be affecting you.

– Nicky Crocker, Geomancer and Earth Healer

The word 'geopathic' is derived from Greek, 'geo' meaning 'the Earth', and 'pathos' meaning 'disease' or 'suffering' and can be translated as 'the suffering of the Earth'. The term 'geopathic stress' (GS) is used to describe negative energies, also known as 'harmful earth rays', which emanate from the Earth and cause discomfort and ill health to those living above. Earth energies can be good, bad, or neutral. 'Bad' energies are often known as 'black ley lines' and may have a significant effect on human well-being.

The concept of GS is not new. Over 4,000 years ago the Chinese recognised destructive earth vibrations that they called 'dragon lines' and warned against building houses on such stressful sites. The Chinese Emperor Kuang Yu (2205–2197 BCE) proclaimed, "No dwelling shall be built until the earth diviners have confirmed the intended building site to be free of earth demons." This geomantic tradition continued and 3,000 years later Chen Su Xiao (d. 1332 CE) explained, "In the subterranean regions there are alternate layers of earth and rock and flowing spring waters. These strata rest upon thousands of vapours which are distributed in tens of thousands of branches, veins and threadlike openings." He said, "The body of the earth is like that of a human being. Ordinary people, not being able to see the veins and vessels which are disposed in order within the body of man, think that it is no more than a lump of solid flesh. Likewise, not being able to see the veins and vessels which are disposed in order under the ground, they think that the earth is just an homogenous mass." These hidden 'veins of the Dragon' carried 'vapours' (Qi or life force) and circulated, like the human bloodstream, removing impurities from the body of the Earth. However, they also deposited curative minerals (crystals) within it, and the currents were reflected in the Earth's atmosphere.[7] In modern times the activities of humankind have exacerbated and distorted what used to be a natural phenomenon, with considerable effect on our well-being.

Research findings

Much of the research on the effects of GS has been carried out in Europe, especially Germany, and in Russia and are not therefore directly accessible in English. One such study goes back to 1929. In collaboration with the Berlin Centre for Cancer Research, German scientist and dowser Baron Gustav von Pohl set out to prove that cancer deaths only occurred in people who had been sleeping in beds positioned above a powerful 'water vein' (underground stream). Baron von Pohl mapped the earth energy lines at Vilsbiburg in Southern Bavaria and compared them to the records at the district hospital. Each of the forty-eight recently recorded cancer deaths in the town had been sleeping above the underground streams mapped by von Pohl. He repeated the procedure in Grafenau in 1930, a town with the lowest cancer incidence in the province, and again found a 100% correlation. The Berlin Centre for Cancer Research accepted Pohl's findings and published the information, positing that earth radiation could be a causative factor in cancer. In a two-year trial, which included over 462,000 measurements and 6,942 tests, Austrian Otto Bergmann found that GS affected blood sedimentation, blood pressure, blood circulation, heartbeat, breathing, skin resistance, and electrical conductivity of muscle points. A search on the Internet reveals many such reports – see the Research Listings at the end of the book – and every dowser or anti-geopathic stress practitioner has a huge fund of anecdotal evidence to draw on.

The Global Matrix Grid

The earth's energy grid is an electromagnetic and geometric structure that acts like a skeleton, or scaffolding for the planet. Great earth circles weave across the planet, as though sacred sites were placed along these lines of force to mark a place as sacred. Energy upwellings, volcanoes and fault lines often match the recorded outline of the grid... Stone circles, pyramids, dolmens and ancient mounds are found on these grids, but it has become clear that natural features such as waterfalls, mountains and volcanoes also link up into subtle geometries.

– Earth Grids: The Secret Patterns of Gaia's Sacred Sites, *Hugh Newman*[8]

Over millions of years, life on Earth evolved with a background magnetic field that varied slightly due to electrical storms, telluric, solar and cosmic activity but nevertheless remained relatively stable. As the Earth rotates on its axis, it creates an electromagnet that generates electrical currents through the molten metals at its core. This creates a, usually beneficial, naturally occurring electromagnetic field on the surface of the planet that oscillates at around 7.83 Hz, closely matching the frequency of the alpha human brainwave. However, the magnetic field of the Earth is non-uniform. In other words, it is stronger in some places than it is in others and can suffer distortion. This field was identified by the physicist WO Schumann in 1952 and became known as 'Schumann waves'. Distortion of this 7.83 Hz level creates a stress that has the potential to weaken the immune system, leading to greater susceptibility to viruses, bacteria, parasites, environmental pollution, degenerative disease, and a wide range of health problems. When NASA built the space shuttle the frequency had to be artificially generated to safeguard the health of the astronauts using it, demonstrating how important it is to human well-being. Since then other equally important wave and geometric patterns have also been identified as forming part of a complex grid around the planet. Where lines cross, considerable disharmony may be generated. Certain 'power spots', however, have a naturally elevated field that was utilised by the ancients for healing and communication with the divine in whatever form that was perceived to be.

The Hartmann Net

The strength of the Earth's magnetic field forms lines of force running north-south and east-west in the shape of a rectangular grid that looks very similar to the lines of latitude and longitude on a map. This grid is called the Hartmann Net. Alternate lines are positively or negatively charged. The lines of force of the Hartmann

Net crossing each other may give rise to GS.

The Curry Grid

A second grid system, the Curry Grid, overlays the Hartmann Net. These naturally generated lines of force meet at an angle creating a diamond-shaped pattern looking rather like an old-fashioned leaded window. The Curry Grid appears to give rise to more geopathic stress than the Hartmann Net. Both can interact with each other, and with stress coming from underground water and fault lines etc.

The Planetary Energetic Grid

The Planetary Energetic Grid is postulated to be formed from the Platonic solids, fundamental shapes identified by the Greek mathematician Pythagoras many centuries ago. These shapes meet at intersecting points to form a matrix which is equivalent to the acupuncture meridians and points on the human body. Bill Becker and Bethe Hagens further developed the work of Ivan P. Sanderson, who had identified the structure of an icosahedron network around the Earth, combining it with the research of a Russian team Goncharov, Morozov and Makarov. Their complex grid was anchored to the north and south axial poles and the Great Pyramid at Giza, Egypt. Intersection points on this grid occur at some of the strongest sacred power places on the planet, but disruption or interruption of the grid can cause severe GS.

The Source

The Earth's energy grid can be thought of as a web that holds or links the Earth together. The energy grid is affected by many influences – electricity, magnetism, light, color, heat, sound and matter. The planetary energy grid operates through certain geometrical patterns that follow a specific symmetry. The grids meet at various intersecting points forming a kind of matrix. This is equivalent to the acupressure points on our bodies. These grid points can be found at some of the strongest power places on the planet.
– www.biogeometry.org

Up until modern times, GS and EMFs were produced mainly from natural sources such as underground watercourses, vortexes and anomalies in the Earth's magnetic or electromagnetic fields or the intersection of the geopathic energy grids surrounding the planet, and the geological fault lines and fractures that may occur naturally. Certain minerals such as iron and oil also raised the stress level. Mines, railway cuttings, tunnels, large buildings with steel-piled foundations, underground cables and utility works, and fracking can all distort the Earth's natural field. However, man-made electromagnetic devices and equipment such as electricity generating stations and substations, cell phones, computers, power lines, underfloor-heating, Wi-Fi and other wireless technology, mobile phone aerials, satellites, surveillance equipment, 'smart meters' and the like have created further distortions with an enormous amount of additional stress. Even the water supply to your home, if it is carried in old-fashioned metal pipes that magnify magnetic waves, may have significant implications for your long-term health and the fertility of the planet and everything on it.

Types of naturally occurring geopathic stress

1. **Underground watercourses:** Watercourses emit a vibration that drains the body's bioenergetic field if encountered for long periods of time. This energy radiates upwards so it makes no difference how deep the water is in the ground, or how many floors above ground a person lives. The effect may be strengthened by the presence of reinforcing rods in a man-made structure.

2. **Earth energy grid systems:** The Earth has a subtle, interpenetrating grid consisting of lines of geopathic or geomagnetic vibrations. These grids go deep into the Earth and high above the planet creating a three-dimensional energy field. The lines convey telluric, magnetic, electric and electromagnetic energies. Intersecting, disturbed or conflicting energy lines can create disequi-

librium or 'hot spots' that may need to be healed. Your hands or feet will tingle when on an energy grid and a dowsing rod or pendulum quickly confirms the flow. Each type of grid intersects with others in the overall system, sometimes to the detriment of those living close to the intersection. These grids have been intensely studied over the last century or so and many are named after their founders: the Hartmann Grid, the Curry Grid, the Benker Grid and so on. Magnetic lines attract, electro lines stimulate and energize, and electromagnetic lines both activate and attract. Ancient peoples had an innate understanding of these telluric energies which could perhaps be described as the Earth's nervous system. Stone circles, temples and the like were inserted into the grid at intersections to activate, amplify, regulate, harmonise and ground the energy flow. The material most often chosen for construction was stone with a high Quartz content.

3. **Vortexes:** Vortexes, an irregular type of geologic energy, also occur naturally. Vortexes are like acupuncture points on the subtle meridian lines of the Earth. These spiral eddies may flow clockwise or anticlockwise in either an outward flow that spirals energy up from the Earth (an electrical vortex) or an inward pull that draws energy from above into the Earth (a magnetic

vortex). Some vortexes are a combination of electromagnetism – 'a vortex within a vortex' – that has both an inward and outward flow. The vortexes and chakras around the globe are linked by energy lines that, when operating properly, create a harmonious but complex geometric pattern (a grid). Disturbances and blockages in the vortexes cause dis-ease elsewhere in the system but crystals can be used to balance the energy and restore equilibrium to the system either at the actual site or through placing crystals on a map.

4. **Geological fractures:** Naturally occurring fault lines are created by pressures within the Earth, especially around tectonic plate junctions, but fault lines can also be caused by blasting or quarrying, and fracking may well have unforeseen GS consequences.

The Effects

The speculative fears of mobile phones being a danger to health in the long run seem to be coming true. A latest study talks about the harmful effects of not just using mobile phones but also the radiation from mobile phone towers. Radiation from mobile phones and towers poses serious health risks, including loss of memory, lack of concentration, disturbance in the digestive system and sleep disturbances. Study on the hazards posed by mobile phones also reported that the damages may not be lethal for humans, but they are worse for birds and insects as well. The studies have attributed the radiation effects to the disappearance of butterflies, bees, insects and sparrows.
– HD Khanna and RK Joshi[9]

As we have seen from the work of Professor Henshaw (see page 23), in those who are electrosensitive, EMFs and GS may create physiological and psychological problems ranging from energy depletion to severe mood swings, hormone imbalances to metabolic syndrome, chronic fatigue to cancer, short-term memory loss or more serious cognitive dysfunction. The adrenal glands can be stuck in permanent 'fight or flight' mode, the immune system may be disabled and the lymphatic system fails. Many aspects of human metabolism, from the ingestion of nutrients to detoxification and the immune response depend on well-functioning bioelectric processes. As the "BioInitiative 2012: A Rationale for Biologically-based Exposure Standards for Low-Intensity Electromagnetic Radiation" report points out: "The stakes are very high. Human beings are bioelectrical systems. Our hearts and brains are regulated by internal bioelectrical signals. Environmental exposures to artificial EMFs may interact with fundamental biological processes in the human body." It goes on to warn:

> In some cases, this may cause discomfort, or sleep disruption, or loss of well-being (impaired mental functioning and impaired metabolism); or sometimes, maybe it is a dread disease like cancer or Alzheimer's disease. It may be interfering with one's ability to become pregnant, or carry a child to full term, or result in brain development changes that are bad for the child. It may be these exposures play a role in causing long-term impairments to normal growth and development of children, tipping the scales away from becoming productive adults. We have good evidence these exposures may damage our health, or that of children of the future who will be born to parents now immersed in wireless exposures.[10]

The report is not scaremongering. As we have seen, the

effects of EMF radiation and GS have been extensively studied in Europe and Russia over the last thirty or more years. This report was prepared by twenty-nine authors from ten countries, ten holding medical degrees, twenty-one PhDs, and three MSc, MA or MPHs. Among the authors were three former presidents of the Bioelectromagnetics Society, and five full members of BEMS. One distinguished author was the Chair of the Russian National Committee on Non-Ionizing Radiation Protection, another a Senior Advisor to the European Environment Agency. The report investigated over 1,800 of the latest studies reporting the bioeffects and adverse health effects of EMFs and wireless technologies. Their conclusion was that:

> Bioeffects are clearly established and occur at very low levels of exposure to electromagnetic fields and radiofrequency radiation. Bioeffects can occur in the first few minutes at levels associated with cell and cordless phone use. Bioeffects may also occur from just minutes of exposure to mobile phone masts (cell towers), Wi-Fi, and wireless utility 'smart' meters that produce whole-body exposure. Chronic base station level exposures can result in illness.[11]
> (See Appendix)

The effects may be particularly significant for children:

> Consistent epidemiologic evidence of an association

between childhood leukemia and exposure to extremely low frequency (ELF) magnetic fields has led to their classification by the International Agency for Research on Cancer as a "possible human carcinogen". Concerns about the potential vulnerability of children to radio frequency (RF) fields have been raised because of the potentially greater susceptibility of their developing nervous systems; in addition, their brain tissue is more conductive, RF penetration is greater relative to head size, and they will have a longer lifetime of exposure than adults.[12]

Evidence for an assumption within the scientific community of the existence of detrimental EMF effects can be found in the most unlikely places. In a 2009 patent application by Stiftelsen University at Bergen, the inventors refer to a previously unrecognised means of intercell communication and state:

> We have also shown that the tunneling nanotubes (TNTs) provide the structural basis for a new type of cell-to-cell communication. TNTs also appear in fixed cells, but they exhibit extreme sensitivity and they are easily destroyed as e.g. prolonged light excitation leads to visible vibrations and rupture. Thus, not only bioactive substances such as drugs but also electromagnetic fields (EMF) such as light and microwaves may compromise TNT-dependent cell-to-cell communication and cause pathological effects in multicel-

lular organisms... we propose to use natural nanotubes as sensors for electromagnetic pollution in order to evaluate both the beneficial and negative effects of drugs and electromagnetic field exposure... A further aspect of the invention relates to a set-up for performing quantitative measurements... which can be employed by manufacturers and institutions wishing to assess the biological effects of electromagnetic fields, for example, the pharmaceutical and medical field, manufacturers of mobile phones, research institutes assessing environmental pollution.[13]

Similarly, geopathic stress can disrupt physiological balance. If your bed is located over a geopathic or underground water line, for instance, insomnia will be the most likely result. You will have difficulty in falling, and remaining, asleep. Waking between 2 and 3am is common as GS reaches a maximum at this time of the night, especially with a full moon. But other chronic health problems such as cancer may well arise.

The most effective action you can take is to move: either to move the bed, a favourite chair and your desk, or, for the worst-case scenario, move house or change your office altogether. But, there are tools which may assist, crystals being among them.

Electromagnetic and Geopathic pollution – symptoms of physiological and psychological distress

The following is a comprehensive list of the reported effects of EMF and GS. It has been culled from many sources but may not be definitive. These symptoms may also be present for reasons other than EMF or geopathic stress.

Sleep disturbances

- Insomnia
- Difficulty in falling asleep
- Difficulty in staying asleep around 3am
- Sleep disorders such as apnoea
- Waking frequently during the night
- Restless sleep
- Nightmares
- Night sweats or night terrors
- Sense of a presence in the room
- Waking too early
- Feeling cold or shivering in bed
- Feeling exceptionally tired on waking
- Sleep is better away from home
- No appetite in the morning

Physical signs and symptoms

- Inability to heal
- Excessive yawning or choking cough
- Nausea

- Drowsiness
- Dizziness
- Weakness
- Cancer
- Autoimmune diseases
- Neurological diseases
- ME
- Headaches
- Blurred vision
- Blackouts
- Irritability
- Fatigue
- Abnormally hot or cold extremities
- Inability to sit for very long
- ADD (Attention Deficit Disorder)
- Miscarriage or failure to conceive
- Sudden infant death syndrome

Physiological disturbances

- Infertility
- Depleted immune system
- Chronic fatigue syndrome
- Constantly feeling vaguely out of sorts and ill at ease
- Increased susceptibility to virus and bacterial infection
- Chronic disease or very slow recovery time from a common illness
- Constant small infections and colds or flu-like

symptoms
- Skin ailments
- Susceptibility to cancer
- Hyper-arousal of the adrenal system
- Neurotransmitter imbalances
- Muscular aches, pains and weakness
- Increase in stress hormones
- Accelerated heartbeat
- Increased breathing rate
- Increased blood sugar
- Hypertension
- Muscle cramps, tension and pain
- Numbness in arms and legs
- Tingling in arms and legs
- Neck pain
- Loss of sex drive
- Temporary impotence (improves away from home)
- Migraine headaches
- Diarrhoea
- Constipation
- Cramping and bloating
- Ulcers
- Irritable bowel
- Weight gain
- Accumulation of abdominal fat
- Overactive thyroid with weight loss
- Diabetes

Psychological disturbances

- Extreme mood swings
- Learning difficulties
- Inappropriate responses to major changes in life situations
- Depression
- Panic attacks
- Paranoia (feeling 'someone is watching me')
- Overwhelming sadness without a cause
- Mood dysfunction, depression and apathy
- Feelings of impending doom
- Constant anxiety without cause
- Sense of helplessness
- Constant negative emotions
- Memory loss
- Lack of concentration
- Irrational thought patterns and confusion
- Aggression
- Problems staying calm
- Insecurity
- Self-confidence problems
- Apathy: lack of interest in doing something
- Decision-making problems

'Random' symptoms

- A formerly clear crystal looks murky in a very short time
- Sick building syndrome
- Cracks in buildings not caused by settlement

- A child or animal is disturbed and cannot settle
- Light bulbs blow frequently
- Electrical apparatus malfunctions
- Constant sharp shocks as though from static electricity
- Batteries and electric items lose their charge very quickly
- Unpleasant or unusual smells
- Cold patches
- There is a history of illnesses such as cancer in previous owners of a property
- Accident blackspot
- The energy feels like walking through treacle
- A property is extremely difficult to sell or changes hands frequently
- Ghosts, out of body experiences and other metaphysical phenomena occur frequently, increasing with prolonged exposure
- Moving house is accompanied by rapid onset of symptoms of relief
- You feel better when away from home

The Six Stages of Geopathic Stress

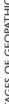

Through many years of hands-on practical research by herself and her colleagues, New Zealand geomancer Nicky Crocker has identified six progressive stages of GS and their accompanying symptoms.[14] She points out that the stages may manifest differently both in timing and severity according to personal sensitivity. In someone who is extremely sensitive the effects may be felt within hours, but for someone less sensitive the subtle symptoms may creep up unnoticed particularly at stage one which then morphs into the progressive stages. These stages have a particularly strong effect on neurotransmitters (chemicals by which a nerve cell communicates with another nerve cell or muscle) and hormone balance which in turn leads to specific symptoms. In Nicky's experience, GS leads to sexual dysfunction, increases the likelihood of illness, and the manifestation of skin ailments and serious illnesses. If the GS never shuts off (i.e. sleeping for 7–8 hours a night in a stressed bed and also working on a GS zone) then these stress hormones produce feelings of anxiety and helplessness.

Oversensitivity to GS has been linked with severe depression, because depressed people have a harder time adapting to the negative side effects of the stress hormone cortisol. As EMFs may contribute to GS, these stages may also correspond to reactions to EMFs.

The six stages of geopathic stress related illness

Stage 1: can occur within hours to 1–2 months. Typical symptoms: 'dis-ease', slow to heal, mood swings, apathy, worry, feeling uncomfortable in bed.

Stage 2: can occur within a few days to several months. Typical symptoms: sleep disorders, nightmares, headaches, fatigue.

Stage 3: can take a few months or several years to occur. Typical symptoms: accelerated heartbeat, hypertension, depression, cramps, anxiety, lack of sex drive.

Stage 4: takes between 1 and 3 years for symptoms to occur. Typical symptoms: diarrhoea, poor digestion, colon irritation, ulcers, irritable bowel syndrome, obesity.

Stage 5: symptoms can take between 3–5 years to occur. Typical symptoms: diabetes, panic attacks, learning difficulties, behaviour problems, ADHD, chronic fatigue, memory problems.

Stage 6: symptoms can occur within 5 years or more, and this stage is associated with a high risk for serious cardiac events and complete suppression of the immune system. Typical symptoms: cancer, cardiovascular events, stroke, diabetes. (Nicky Crocker)

Stage 1: Negative feelings and strange sensations

Although there are few physical symptoms at this stage, neurotransmitter imbalance has already occurred and neurotransmitters such as serotonin are inhibited resulting in:

- Constant low-level bacterial and viral infections
- Slow recovery from common illnesses such as colds and flu
- Mood dysfunction and apathy
- Feeling uncomfortable in your bed, favourite armchair, or workplace without any particular reason
- Unpleasant sensations
- Flabbiness
- Worry
- Unreasonable sadness

Stage 2: Negative emotions and sleep disorders

This stage is typically characterized by continued neurotransmitter imbalance that leads to sleep disorders and negative emotional effects. Constant inhibition of neurotransmitters such as serotonin, GABA (Gama amino butyric acid) and norepinephrine (or noradrenaline, a hormone secreted by the adrenal medulla, increasing blood pressure and heart rate) can lead to insomnia, restless sleep and waking up tired. Those symptoms, which may be intermittent, can disrupt people's lifestyle and lead to symptoms such as weakness and drowsiness. Negative emotions occur when there is a decrease in serotonin or GABA and can cause feelings of depression, anxiety, and impending doom. It can affect work relationships, and create family conflicts.

- Difficulty falling asleep
- Difficulty staying asleep
- Waking too early
- Restless sleep
- Waking frequently
- Nightmares
- Night sweats
- Feeling cold or shivering in bed
- Impending doom
- Drowsiness
- Dizziness
- Weakness
- Headaches
- Irritability
- Fatigue
- Feeling depressed
- Anxiety
- Lack of appetite in the morning

Stage 3: Stress hormones

This is when major symptoms occur. The body starts to actively respond to the natural radiation threat. Having experienced constant intense negative emotions (stage 2) and continual long-term GS influence, the brain responds by initiating over 1,400 physiological responses, including activating the hypothalamic-pituitary-adrenal (HPA) system. The hypothalamus sends signals to the sympathetic nervous system which triggers the production and release of the stress hormone cortisol. Cortisol is very important in the marshalling system throughout the body, including the heart, lungs, circulation, metabolism, and immune system. The HPA system also releases catecholamines from the adrenal glands in response to stress and the 'fight-or-flight' hormones dopamine, norepinephrine, and epinephrine. Epinephrine (adrenalin) raises the heart rate, breathing rate, blood pressure, and the amount of sugar in the blood. This can lead to symptoms including: fatigue and weakness, muscle and bone loss, moodiness or depression, hormone imbalance, and suppression of the immune system. In short bursts, elevated adrenalin is not damaging or dangerous. But sustained at high levels over a period of time, it can be very harmful. Long-term over-arousal and excessive flow of this hormone will eventually lead to physiological and psychological distress.

- Accelerated human heartbeat
- Increased breathing rate
- Increased blood sugar
- Hypertension
- Depression

- Muscle cramps tension, pain
- Numbness in arms and legs
- Tingling in arms and legs
- Neck pain
- Anxiety
- Loss of sex drive
- Lack of interest in sex
- Helplessness
- Temporary impotence
- Migraine headaches

Stage 4: Digestive system disorders

It takes one to three years for symptoms to occur in this stage. As the human organism tries to adapt by producing and activating more hormones, increasing blood pressure, and raising blood sugar levels to sustain energy, it depletes the body's energy reserves, gradually weakening the organism, upsetting homeostasis (a state of equilibrium in which all body systems are working and interacting harmoniously) and affects the internal organs, leaving the body vulnerable to diseases. Diseases of the stomach and intestines are often linked to GS because the blood has to leave these organs and move to muscles. Cortisol and DHEA (dehydroepiandrosterone, produced in the body and converted into male and female hormones) work as a team to get people through prolonged GS's effects. DHEA is the most abundant hormone in the bloodstream. It appears to balance the effects of cortisol, improving the body's ability to cope.

DHEA also provides the base material for the production of many other hormones including oestrogen, progesterone, and testosterone. But an imbalance can result in chronic symptoms:

- Raised blood pressure
- Increased blood sugar
- Diarrhoea
- Constipation
- Cramping
- Bloating
- Stomach ache
- Ulcers
- Irritable Bowel Syndrome
- Accumulation of abdominal fat
- Weight gain
- Hyperactivity of the thyroid gland
- Fatigue
- Bone loss
- Loss of muscle mass
- Decreased sex drive
- Impaired immune function
- Mental problems
- Memory impairment
- Lack of energy
- Heart and blood vessel diseases
- Depression
- Increased susceptibility to stroke and cancer

Stage 5: On constant alert

In this stage, the body has run out of its reserve of body energy and immunity, and symptoms can occur within 3–5 years. Mental, physical and emotional resources suffer heavily. A few years' overreaction to GS overloads the brain with powerful hormones that are intended only for short-term duty in emergency situations. The cumulative effect is damage and death of brain cells. Catecholamines suppress activity in areas at the front of the brain concerned with memory, concentration, inhibition, and rational thought. Stress hormones divert blood glucose from the brain, and hypothalamus function is diminished. The hypothalamus continues to signal to the adrenals to produce cortisol and the increased cortisol production exhausts the stress mechanism, leading to chronic fatigue and anxiety. Cortisol also interferes with serotonin activity, furthering the depressive effect. Prolonged high cortisol levels lead to high blood sugar that may develop into diabetes. The adrenals become depleted, leading to decreased GS tolerance, progressive mental and physical exhaustion, illness and collapse. It affects the major organs and systems. The body becomes more susceptible to infections, minor and major.

- Damaged immune system
- Inability to heal
- Increased susceptibility to infection
- Brain cell damage

- Loss of concentration at work and at home
- Learning problems
- Damaged cardiovascular and respiratory systems, kidney, muscles, and joints
- Inappropriate responses to major changes in life situations
- Inability to sit for very long
- Behavioural problems
- Aggression
- Problems staying calm
- Insecurity
- Self-confidence problems
- Panic attacks
- Emotional problems (anxiety, depression, and exhaustion)
- Diabetes
- Memory problems
- Lack of interest in doing anything
- Decision-making problems
- ADD (Attention Deficit Disorder)
- Chronic Fatigue

Stage 6: Immune system collapse

The human organism eventually loses all its resistance to the prolonged effects of GS, and this stage is associated with complete suppression of the immune system and a high risk of serious cardiac events. Symptoms can occur within 5 years or more. Adrenal exhaustion creates depletion of energy reserves and loss of resilience to GS may take place slowly or rapidly. This means the immune system and the body's ability to resist diseases may be almost totally eliminated making the body more susceptible to everything from colds and flu to cancer – a number of studies have shown that subjects under GS have low white blood cell counts and are particularly vulnerable to infections and diseases. Recent research has also made it clear that hyper-arousal of the adrenal system is a causative factor in coronary and arterial diseases. People who have relatively low levels of the neurotransmitter serotonin produce more of certain immune proteins (cytokines), which in high amounts cause inflammation and damage to cells. Cortisol levels also appear to play a role in the accumulation of abdominal fat. This can lead to greater risk factors for heart attack, heart rhythm abnormalities and stroke. Continually raised cortisol levels lead to suppression of the immune system through increased production of interleukin-6 (an immune system messenger).

- Immune system failure
- Cardiovascular diseases
- Cancer
- Heart attack
- Arthritis
- Kidney disorders
- Cell disorders
- Allergies

- Skin diseases: psoriasis, eczema, hives and acne
- Bronchial asthma
- Stroke
- Infertility and miscarriages
- Pneumonia
- Periodontal disease
- High blood pressure
- Increased heart rate
- Constricted arteries
- Arrhythmia
- Artery-clogging blood clots
- Low white blood cell count
- Increase in the production of cholesterol
- Decrease in the body's ability to remove cholesterol
- Overactive B-cells
- Defective regulation by T-cells

Fortunately all these stages, even the most serious, can be reversed by removing yourself from the source of the GS, or by taking steps to counteract it as this brief case history from Nicky shows:

Energy Bombs

I have a lady whose lower part of her bed had GS running through it and I asked her where her two cats slept. She informed me they slept right at the end of her bed, which was also where she was having problems in her legs. We put one of my 'Energy Defusers' (I call them Energy Bombs and they are designed to help calm and neutralise the effects of GS) and she noticed that the cats stopped sleeping on that same position where the 'bombs' were directly under the bed. Interesting!

After 6 months she noticed they started to sleep back on the bed. So I suggested she recharge the crystals in the sun or full moon, and they stopped sleeping there again. She is thrilled and also her legs improved.

Nicky's story shows the importance of cleansing and recharging crystals when they are part of anti-geopathic stress tools (see page 134 for the full version of Nicky's case history and the crystals she uses).

Photographing the Fields

All living creatures generate and emit subtle radiation. Photons of light, electromagnetic frequencies, heat, sound, and scent are all emitted from our bodies in direct relationship to our internal state. This subtle system of exchange can be photographed with a Kirlian camera. Kirlian photography, named after Russian electrician Semyon Davidovich Kirlian, was discovered by accident. Kirlian photographic techniques use high voltage, high frequency, ultra low current, electrical fields. In travelling through and reacting with the body's complex systems, this influx of electrical energy amplifies and makes visible the body's biological energy exchange by producing a corona of multi-frequency energy waves – from low infrared to well past the visible spectrum – which can be photographed. Kirlian photography graphically illustrates the effect of GS and EMFs on the human bioenergetic field.

In this example photograph, an electrically sensitive person held a mobile phone that was switched on but not connected. As can be seen, the auric field literally fell apart. When a Black Tourmaline was taped to the phone, the field regenerated although still had some anomalies.

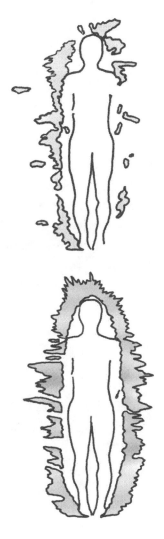

(1) Bioenergy field with mobile phone switched on but not transmitting or receiving and (2) aura with Black Tourmaline protector on the mobile phone.

Recognising When You're at Risk

So, how do you recognise geopathically stressed areas or whether you are suffering from EMF sensitivity? Well apart from their noticeable effect on health and well-being in those who are sensitive, both can be dowsed for – and you will probably have identified several symptoms if you are at risk. You may also feel it in the environment. The energy is heavy and 'sticky'. I always describe it as 'walking through treacle' but you may simply feel the need to open a window because you are yawning a lot and the air feels stale. Or you may notice that you feel distinctly worse after being in a particular place for any length of time.

There are immediate pointers for GS. Trees tend to grow well on one side and noticeably less well on the other. The trunk will twist to get away from the stress. There may be a line of stunted growth through a crop. As we saw from Nicky Crocker's case history above, animals – cats rather than dogs – are attracted to areas of geomagnetic stress and will often sleep on a toxic line with resultant diseases such as cancers, kidney or liver failure. Babies and young children tend to try to escape from geopathic lines, squidging up in a corner of their cot, toddlers and older children sleepwalk or climb into their parents' bed to escape from the effects. If the parents' bed is on the line they themselves may well sleep at an angle to avoid it and will suffer from insomnia and restlessness. Older children exhibit behavioural problems and constant low-level illnesses, as may the adults.

If you see a dead or dying tree leaning at an angle and covered in ivy, a mass of ants and bees or termites, and a line of stunted growth through crops or trees that flower but do not bear fruit, and a crack on a building, aligned with an area of quarrying or other earth disturbance, a high water table or an underground watercourse or metal pipes, and the inhabitants of that building are diseased or chronically sick, or a combination of the above, then you can be pretty certain that the building is sitting on a geopathic stress line.

Also, do bear in mind that geopathic stress is being created all the time. If you live in a city, or elsewhere, that has building or construction work such as tunnelling or deep foundation pile-driving, geopathic stress may being newly created in a formerly stress free zone. Existing zones may change. When repair work was done on the substation close to me after it had been struck by lightning I had to reposition all my crystals to accommodate the amped up GS, and when the village Wi-Fi came on stream, more crystals were needed, for instance. It is a good idea to dowse at regular intervals to check, or keep a close eye on the behaviour of your pets.

However, don't get too fixated on the idea of GS or you may create something that wasn't there in the first place. A client of mine shared a house with a healer who had an arthritic hip. The healer insisted it must be down to GS but several dowsers all confirmed that there was no geopathic stress affecting the house, which suggested it had another basis. The healer nevertheless maintained there could be no other explanation. Eventually a dowser found a line – right through the corner of the room where the healer slept, cutting across the bed at the level of his hip. "There I knew it," he said. My client wasn't convinced and still believes that the healer manufactured the line from his insistence that GS must be the cause rather than facing his own issues. She felt increasingly unwell in the house and moved out, but not before discovering eleven different anti-GS devices, several running off electricity and therefore generating EMFs, placed at random all over the house – which was probably what was affecting my client as she had become extremely energy-sensitive. The devices could have been beneficial had there been GS, but as there was not the effect was detrimental, disturbing her previously balanced and healthy energy field. The healer had placed them 'in case' but, unsurprisingly, his hip did not improve. So, be careful what you wish for, you may inadvertently create exactly what you are trying to avoid.

Fortunately, as I have found, crystals can create subtle energetic grids that protect you from the effects of EMFs and GS and which, as long as they are cleansed regularly, support healthy energy fields, instilling beneficial bioenergy patterns and easing the physiological and psychological symptoms and effects. These tools have not yet been researched to scientifically acceptable standards but there is sufficient anecdotal evidence in the form of reports from users to support their effects. In this book you will find crystals to assist yourself at various levels (see Part II).

Counteracting the effects

There are five major ways in which protecting yourself from EMF and GS can be approached with crystals:

Approach 1: Shield

This method works well if you have already healed, or have avoided, the detrimental effects of EMFs and GS. A shielding crystal surrounds the outer edge of your bioenergy field with a protective coating and does not let the EMF or GS through into your inner space. Similarly, crystals can be placed next to an EMF source to shield it or on a GS line to deflect it.

Approach 2: Support

Crystals can strengthen your bioenergy field and align it with your physical body, bringing them into harmony and stimulating your immune system to heal and defend itself against detrimental energies.

Approach 3: Transmute

Crystals can transmute toxic energies into beneficial ones, preventing damage in the first place. The crystals act like a voltage converter, changing the frequency and adapting it as necessary.

Approach 4: Ground

Crystals help you to anchor your energies to the Earth, grounding you and strengthening the lower chakras so that you are more resistant to the toxic effects of GS or EMFs. They also ground the energy of EMF or GS sources. Being earthed means that you, or your space, discharge EMFs into the ground.

Approach 5: Negative ions

Ions (from the Greek 'wanderer') are electronically charged atoms or molecules that exist throughout our environment. Ions can be positive or negative. Negatively charged ions stimulate the body's defensive mononuclear phagocyte system, a network of cells that help filter out the dead and toxic. An important part of the larger immune system, it helps maintain healthy organ function and blood chemistry. Negative ions assist the body to repair cellular damage and a strong negative ion field can help to prevent initial damage. Certain crystals such as Amethyst, Zeolite and Tourmaline create negative ions from moisture in the air and build a shielding field with them. This is especially helpful in areas affected by power lines that create harmful positive corona ion streams.

And How Do Crystals Help?

We discovered that when you add a quartz crystal oscillator to the circuit, it starts polarizing to your unique bioenergy field signature. Crystals have the property of being able to stabilize and amplify our energy fields or any energy fields.
– Joe Hall, www.consumerhealth.org

The mineral content and the internal structure of a crystal itself can have a potent effect. Shungite, Shieldite and Fulgarite, for instance, are constructed from 'buckyballs', tiny fullerenes that are getting science very excited. They can absorb and keep pollutants, energetic or substance-based, contained within their hollow structure. They act like a holding pen for EMFs. The effect may be synergistic: mineral and structure combined. Shungite is carbon-based, as is Graphite, and carbon readily filters and absorbs pollutants. So, it is not surprising that Diamond, created under tremendous pressure from pure carbon, is an excellent, if expensive, shield against EMFs. All crystals are formed from minerals that have specific properties: boron absorbs, iron can deflect or attract, silica conducts and so on, and these properties are passed to the crystals of which they are an integral part.

Structure is significant in the Zeolite family which includes Heulandite, Klinoptilolith, Thomsonite, Scolecite, Stilbite, Natrolite and Pollucite. These microporous minerals are used extensively in industry as absorbents and catalysts. They are known as molecular-sieves. Their crystal lattice is a net that has 'spaces' that can trap impurities or filter particles, and they can also exchange molecules such as ions. A powerful, conventional, anti-cancer chemotherapy drug is made from Klinoptilolith. 'Zeolite', based on the zeolite mineral clinoptilolite (Klinoptilolith), is now being marketed as a potent 'alternative treatment' anti-cancer tool and the Internet is flooded with anecdotal evidence as to the effectiveness and potential side effects (see Resources page 259).

The resonance of crystal fields and how they entrain with and harmonise other fields is another clue as to how crystals can help. Especially as the human body is, to a large extent, crystalline with millions of crystals being present in the body in the brain, blood and so on. Crystals have a perfect geometric molecular structure that is coherent and stable, each part replicating the other. They are like holograms that have a very low incidence of entropy – a gradual, and natural, decline into disorder. Human bodies have a very high level of entropy, which means our energetic vibrations can be easily disrupted by internal or external factors. The stable, low entropy state of healing crystals can entrain – that is match – our frequency to theirs, returning our vibrations to a coherent bio-resonant state. This 'perfect state' is one of the reasons why crystals can help with EMF or GS disruption. The stable, organised, coherent field of a crystal is in direct contrast to an EMF or GS field, which is chaotic and disorganised. Put an organised field into a disorganised one and the two will entrain back into the most stable form, an organised field.

In part, however, the answer to how crystals help could be due to colour. Black is a colour that absorbs, and some of the most effective protective and transmuting stones are black, Shungite and Black Tourmaline for instance. Orange and red crystals such as Red Jasper and Triplite create an active, beneficial field to counter a negative. But the answer may well lie elsewhere. It is my belief that entrainment and bioscalar waves are what make crystals such an efficient healing, transmutation and shielding mechanism (see below). Crystals have their own bio- and electromagnetic field and beneficial scalar waves. The subtle electrically charged bioenergy patterns that crystals carry restore the disharmonious resonance of EMFs and GS back into harmony so that they are better dealt with by the human body, and support the body in its bioprocesses. The positive field balances out and negates the negative one.

At this point in time, there is no specific answer to the mechanism by which crystals work their magic. All you can do is try it and see. However, you need to ensure that the crystal is compatible with your energy field before using it. Dowsing or your intuition will assist in your choices (see page 93).

How crystals may help:

Crystals can compensate for the detrimental effects of EMFs and GS on your body, harmonising and rebalancing your energy field and that of your environment so that you have more resistance to the effects of geo- and electropathogens. Crystals also heal sick building syndrome.

Crystals can create an energetic net to transmute the detrimental energy field through entrainment with a beneficial one (more of that later).

Crystals help you to stay earthed and grounded. If you have your feet firmly on the planet and your lower chakras are open and clear, you will be much more resistant to noxious or toxic GS and EMFs.

Harmonising the flow

That stones can alter the flow of telluric energy has been known since ancient times as the needles of stone inserted in stone circles and temples show. These stones usually have a high silica-rich Quartz content, and silica both discharges, stores and generates energy. Needles of stone either brought earth energies to the surface or diverted their course, or drew cosmic energy down to Earth. These ancient constructions were not randomly placed on the landscape, they were sited where they could control the energies and hold the balance between active – positive – currents, and passive – negative – currents, harmonising the environment.

Fifteen hundred years ago a traditional Chinese medical doctor, Sun Simiao, was asked what principles were used to cure illnesses. His answer was based on maintaining balance between the macrocosm and the microcosm:

If one is skilled at talking about Heaven, one must substantiate it in the human realm; if one is skilled at talking about humans, one must also root it in Heaven. In Heaven, there are four seasons and five phases; winter cold and summer heat alternate with each other. When this cyclical revolution is harmonious, it forms rain; when it is angry, wind; when it congeals, frost and snow; when it stretches out, rainbows. These are the constancies of Heaven and Earth. When the constancies are lost, if qi and essence steam upward, they cause heat in the body; if they are blocked, they cause cold; if they are bound, tumors and excrescences; if they sink, abscesses; if they scatter wildly, panting and shortness of breath; and if they are exhausted, scorching and withering... When one extends this analogy to apply to Heaven and Earth, it is also likewise... Uprighted boulders and thrust-up earth are the tumors and excrescences of Heaven and Earth. Collapsing mountains and caved-in ground are the abscesses of Heaven and Earth. Scattered winds and violent rain are the panting and shortness of breath of Heaven and Earth. Dried-up streams and parched marshes are the scorching and withering of Heaven and Earth. An excellent physician guides... with medicinals and lancing stones and rescues with needles and prescriptions... Thus, the human body has illnesses that can be cured, and Heaven and Earth have calamities that can be dispersed.[15]

In other words, if the planet and the cosmos hold a balance, then the human body will do so too. As can be seen, one of the tools the Chinese doctor recommended was 'lancing stones'. The equivalent of which today would be needles of stone inserted into the Earth to release negative energies or to attract positive ones and to maintain the balance. Or crystals placed on the body to energetically correct imbalances. When placed on a source of detrimental energy, crystals can harmonise the energies so that they are no longer toxic or a source of disturbance to your own energy field. The positive, coherent field neutralising and harmonising a detrimental, disorganised one. However, it is essential to hold the intention that the beneficial field will be the stronger and will entrain the negative into harmony.

Similarly, for many centuries human beings used

stone in their buildings – especially those of a sacred nature – not only for its sturdy constructional qualities but also because the effect of those stones was understood. Stately homes and large farmhouses were anchored with large blocks of stone at the corners. This stone often came from the fields or local quarries and had high silica (Quartz) content. Despite the fact that silica is a semi-conductor much used in the production of electro-magnetic creating products, such as computers, silica has a beneficial field that harmonises EMF energies. Although silica is said to slide into resonance with EMFs, it does so in a way that is healing and protective, harmonising the energy. Silica also harmonises and deflects geopathic stress, causing the detrimental energies to flow around the building rather than through it – something you can mimic today by placing large blocks of suitable stone at the corner of your home. Similarly, many buildings employed Marble, another silica-rich stone, to harmonise or deflect noxious energies. Iron-rich stones such as Hematite, Magnetite or Pyrite also ground and correct energy imbalances.

And finally, as all crystal workers know, these powerful beings can bring your energy field into balance, restoring harmony and homeostasis to your body. They carry the resonance of their component minerals and have their own specific frequency with which your energy field can entrain. Wearing crystals or carrying them on your person makes an enormous difference to how your immune system copes with GS and EMF and how your whole body-mind-spirit functions.

Entrainment

No matter how small their size, crystals emit a subtle energy that links with all other crystals of their type so that the cumulative effect is vast. Entrainment is a subtle energetic interaction. In physics it is defined as the synchronization of two or more rhythmic cycles, but in crystal work it can be seen as a sympathetic resonance between two vibrational fields. In conventional entrainment a smaller energetic field takes on the characteristics of a larger field but this can work both ways, the larger field takes on the characteristics of the smaller especially when directed by intention. Time and distance have no relevance here. Research has shown that the brainwaves of a healer and the recipient synchronise, or resonate no matter how far the distance by which they are separated.[16] Quantum physics has demonstrated that simultaneous transfer of energy is possible. A particle can be in one place and in another *at the same time* and thought can have an instantaneous effect over vast distances. A crystal's pulsing energy field has perfect equilibrium and its sympathetic resonance stabilizes a larger field through energetic synchronisation. This resonance property is used to send healing and rebalancing to a human body, a specific site or the matrix grid through the placement of crystals around the body or a site, or on maps and diagrams to restore balance that is then energetically transferred to the larger energy field.

Such entrainment can be heightened by intention – the power of thought.

Scalar waves

Everything is energy and that everything vibrates at different frequencies. Bio-scalar energy is a unique form of energy that can be harnessed and directed into solid objects or bodies placed in its field.
– Kalon Prensky

Scalar waves are found throughout the universe and within our physical bodies. Bioscalar wave energy exists at the microscopic level in the nucleus of an atom or a cell and creates a bioenergetic source more powerful than DNA, cellular matrixes and other physiological processes. Whilst some bioscalar waves may be viewed as harmful, beneficial bioscalar waves have been shown to energize the extracellular matrix of the body and protect against electromagnetic emanations and geopathic stress that would otherwise detrimentally affect cells and tissue. They activate the meridians and facilitate healing at the energetic interface between spirit and matter.[17] It is probable that all healing crystals have this energy within their matrix, and that their crystalline structure actually produces bioscalar energy. If, as Lilli Botchis asserts, "when the human body enters a scalar wave field, the electromagnetic field of the individual becomes excited [and] this catalyzes the mind/body complex to return to a more optimal state that is representative of its original, natural, electrical matrix form,"[18] we can see how a crystal with its optimal energy pattern might operate on the human and planetary energy body.

In physics, a scalar wave is defined as a standing wave that has no GPS coordinates and is not dependant on time or space. In healing or shielding terms, this means that the "active spinning vortices composed of quantities of energy that interact with all non-physical dimensions including consciousness" can be anywhere and everywhere instantaneously and simultaneously. Like two piano strings with the same tone, energy can be exchanged and aligned through resonance and vibration. Many if not all crystals generate scalar waves. Given what we have already discovered about the Earth's matrix grid, a quick look at current definitions of scalar waves shows us that they are intelligent and proactive and indicates how they might function in crystal healing, and EMF and GS protection:

A scalar wave is *non-linear*, not electromagnetic, and exists in multiple dimensions beyond time or space. That means they do not decay with time or distance from their source. Scalar waves can interact with all matter including electro-magnetism but since they are non-linear and hyperspatial, they... must be detected and measured indirectly... A scalar transmitter can wirelessly send power to a receiver through any obstacle... [even] a Faraday Cage or a metal box, and a receiver can receive power far away. During the process of transmission and reception they can magnify power.

(www.homeotronics.com)

A Scalar Wave is not a single wave but a result of the interaction (interference) of multiple waves of very high frequency which seem to modulate and encode each other in a harmonious holistic complexity, similar to a hologram. The resulting multi-dimensional standing wave pattern emanates out of a fixed source point (a healer) [or crystal] and can be received and decoded by a similar resonant quantum-connected receiver point (recipient)... This causes vibrational ripples in the Morphogenic Field of the Cosmic Unified Field. (www.keylonticdictionary.org)

Amping up the protection

I have found that adding crystal and flower essences to EMF and anti-GS crystals and grids amps up the power enormously. The crystals hold the signature of the essence for a considerable time and the synergy is greater than the power of the individual items. I have used Petaltone essence Clear2Light to clear and recharge my crystals for many years and could not work without it. Petaltone EMF essence works exceptionally well when placed on clear Quartz or Selenite and left in place, as does the Australian Bush Flower's Electromagnetic essence. Petaltone Temple Flame and Clear2Light proved to be extremely efficient at clearing and re-energizing Shungite and other crystals. Sue and Simon Lilly of Green Man Tree essences make a Shungite gem essence and the excellent Shield 1 spray or essence (a combination of Quartz Buckyball, Shungite, Preseli Bluestone, Galena, Mandala 14, Linear Water and The Merlin). It was created in response to a request from Japan following the Fukushima disaster (see Resources for these and other essence companies).

The Protective Chakras

The chakras act as linkage points between the physical and subtle bodies, and between those bodies and the Earth, mediating the flow of energy between the two. Their function is not limited to this activity but it is extremely useful in protecting the physical body from the effects of GS and EMFs, especially as the chakras also have subtle connections with the Earth and the cosmos. One of the most helpful things you can do for yourself is to strengthen your grounding through the Earth Star and base chakras by sending a root deep down into the centre of the Earth (see page 88) and keeping the chakras open – unless you are in an area of severe geopathic stress, in which case protecting your Earth Star may be necessary until you reach a place where the energies are more harmonious. These chakras are vitally important in maintaining a sense of safety and security, and overcoming fear. Having this grounding cord in place at all times helps you to feel safe. Keeping your dantien charged up gives you a reserve of energy on which to draw, helping to overcome the fatigue induced by EMFs and GS. Placing crystals on the chakras helps to strengthen your own energy field which is then better equipped to resist the ill effects. Certain chakras, which are described in detail here, have a particularly important part to play in EMF and GS protection, but the location of all the chakras can be seen in the illustration below.

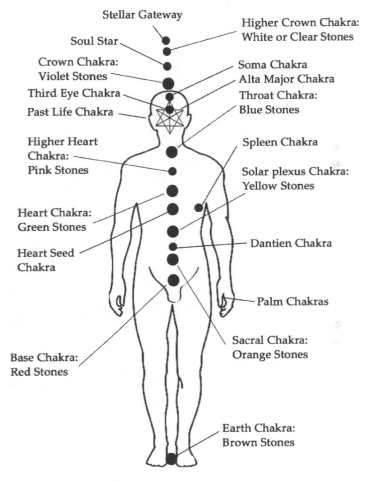

Stellar Gateway

Higher Crown Chakra:
White or Clear Stones

Soul Star

Crown Chakra:
Violet Stones

Soma Chakra
Alta Major Chakra

Third Eye Chakra

Throat Chakra:
Blue Stones

Past Life Chakra

Higher Heart
Chakra:
Pink Stones

Spleen Chakra

Solar plexus Chakra:
Yellow Stones

Heart Chakra:
Green Stones

Heart Seed
Chakra

Dantien Chakra

Palm Chakras

Base Chakra:
Red Stones

Sacral Chakra:
Orange Stones

Earth Chakra:
Brown Stones

Crystals and the Chakras

GS and EMF protective chakras

Earth Star (beneath your feet)

Area: Everyday reality and groundedness.

Physiology: The physical body, electrical systems of the body and the sensory organs.

Effect: Earth Star imbalances or disruptions lead to discomfort in your physical body, feelings of helplessness and ungroundedness accompanied by an inability to function practically in the world. An out of balance Earth Star picks up adverse environmental factors such as GS, 'black' ley lines and toxic pollutants. It is highly sensitive to EMF pollution as it governs the electrical systems of the body and is your connection to GS through the soles of your feet with their many nerve endings. When this chakra is functioning well you are grounded and comfortable in incarnation with a well-functioning immune system.

Typical dis-eases are lethargic: ME, arthritis, cancer, muscular disorders, depression, psychiatric disturbances, autoimmune diseases.

Base (base of your spine/perineum)

Area: Basic survival instincts and security issues.

Physiology: Gonads, adrenals, veins, lower back, rectum, lower extremities, lymph system, skeleton system (teeth and bones), immune system, prostate gland, kidney, bladder and elimination system, sense of smell.

Effect: Your base chakra is linked to your core and your

connection to Earth. If it is affected by GS or EMFs your immune system cannot protect you. Imbalances or disruptions in this chakra lead to insecurity and feelings of anger, impotence and frustration. Lacking bioenergetic balance, you will be ungrounded and may be unwilling to accept your connection to the Earth, feeling uncomfortable in your physical body and seeking escape. When it is functioning well you are confident and self-assertive, and able to deal effectively with environmental stresses.

Typical dis-eases are constant low level or flare up suddenly: stiffness in joints, chronic lower back pain, renal, reproductive or rectal disorders such as fluid retention or constipation (diarrhoea if stuck open), varicose veins or hernias, the extremes of bipolar disorder, glandular disturbances, personality and anxiety disorders, autoimmune diseases.

Sacral (navel) (slightly below your waist)
Area: Creativity, fertility and acceptance of yourself as a sexual being.
Physiology: Testes, ovaries, uterus, lumbar and pelvic region, spleen, large intestine, immune system, kidneys, gallbladder, bladder and elimination system, the sense of taste.
Effect: Imbalances or disruptions in this chakra lead to infertility and blocked creativity. A component of your core energy system and your ability to manifest, it also assists you to hold your boundaries steady. When it is

functioning well you are creative and enlivened.

Typical dis-eases are toxic and psychosomatic: PMT and muscle cramps, reproductive blockages or diseases, impotence, infertility, allergies, addictions, eating disorders, diabetes, liver or intestinal dysfunction – irritable bowel, chronic back pain, urinary infections.

Dantien (on top of the sacral, just beneath navel)
Area: The powerpoint.
Physiology: Autonomic nervous and energy-conductive systems, regulation of the functioning of internal organs and involuntary processes such as breathing and heartbeat. Sensory impulses to the brain.
Effect: An adjunct to the sacral chakra and the point of balance for the physical body, the dantien is where Qi, life force, is stored and your body earthed. This is your core energy source. Disruption here means that Qi cannot circulate efficiently and is not replenished and the autoimmune system cannot function. If the dantien is too open, energy is constantly drained. When it is functioning well you are energized and power-full.
Typical dis-eases relate to physical function and energy utilisation: nervous system dysfunctions, autoimmune diseases, cardiac problems, high blood pressure, orthostatic hypotension, palpitations, adrenal overload, chronic fatigue, ME, Raynaud's, Parkinson's, digestive problems, diabetes, light-headedness, powerlessness, feeling ill at ease in incarnation.

Higher heart (thymus) (between the heart and the throat)

Area: Compassion and safety.

Physiology: The psychic and physical immune systems, thymus gland, lymphatic system, elimination and purification organs.

Effect: If this chakra is disturbed your psychic and physical immune systems will not be able to function, and it will not be able to protect your physical heart. If it is functioning well you are psychically and physically strong, and feel safe in incarnation.

Typical dis-eases follow those of the heart, arteriosclerosis together with viral infections and immune system disorders, tinnitus, epilepsy.

Soma chakra (above the third eye, at the hairline)

Area: Spiritual connection.

Physiology: The connection point between the subtle energetic systems and the physical, etheric and light bodies.

Effect: This chakra is where your subtle bodies, including the lightbody, attach themselves to the physical. When this chakra is stuck open it is all too easy for you to float out of your physical body, and such disconnection leaves you open to EMF or GS invasion. If it is functioning well you can safely explore the spiritual dimensions of life.

Typical dis-eases are autistic and disconnected or dyspraxic and may include Down's Syndrome, autism and ADHD, chronic fatigue, delusional states.

Alta Major (inside the skull, the access point is at the base of the skull)

Area: Accelerating and expanding consciousness.

Physiology: The subtle and physical endocrine systems, hippocampus, hypothalamus, pineal and pituitary glands; brain function, the cerebellum and voluntary muscle movements, the medulla oblongata controlling breathing, heart rate and blood pressure; occipital area and the optic nerve, throat, spine, sleeping patterns.

Effect: If the alta major is functioning well your subtle endocrine system harmonises the subtle bodies with the physical. You will have a strong sense of direction in life and a well-functioning immune system. If the chakra is disturbed or disconnected, you will feel disorientated, open to paranoid delusions – which will feel like reality – and energetic sensing of subtle disturbances in the environment around you. You may feel like you've been taken over by something outside yourself.

Typical diseases are ancestral, karmic or those of disorientation: metabolic dysfunction, eye problems, floaters, cataracts, migraine, headaches and feelings of confusion, 'dizziness' or 'floatiness', loss of sense of purpose and spiritual depression, fear, terror, adrenaline rush.

Crown (top of your head)

Area: Spiritual communication and awareness.

Physiology: Pituitary, hypothalamus, brain, spine, central nervous system, hair, subtle energy bodies.

Effect: If the crown chakra is disturbed you will be

disconnected from your spiritual self and from cosmic energies. Spiritual interference or possession may result, and metabolic imbalances are common. If it is functioning well you express yourself as a spiritual being and attain unity consciousness.

Typical dis-eases arise out of disconnection: metabolic syndrome, 'unwellness' with no known cause, nervous system disturbances, electromagnetic and environmental sensitivity, depression, dementia, ME, insomnia or excessive sleepiness, 'biological clock' disturbances such as jet lag.

The palm chakras

There are also chakras in the palms of your hands that can help you to select crystals or establish where energy lines run. To open these chakras, put your palms together and then pull them apart, push them together again and continue until you can feel a ball of energy build up in your palms, which will pulsate. To close them, hold your hands under running water, or place them firmly together.

To open a chakra

Picture the chakra opening like the petals of a flower until the chakra is fully open and energetic.

To close a chakra

Picture the petals closing back into a tight ball.

The grounding root

Keeping your Earth Star chakra open and grounded into the centre of the planet assists in deterring the effects of GS and helps you to be comfortable in incarnation. The simplest way to do this is with a visualization:

- Picture the Earth Star chakra about a foot beneath your feet opening like the petals of a water lily (you can also place a Smoky Quartz or Smoky Elestial Quartz at your feet to assist).
- Feel two roots growing from the soles of your feet down to meet the Earth Star where they meet.
- The two roots twine together and pass down through the Earth Star going deep into the earth. They pass through the outer mantle, down past the solid crust and deep into the molten magma.
- When the entwined roots have passed through the magma, they reach the big iron crystal ball at the centre of the planet.
- The roots hook themselves around this ball, holding you firmly in incarnation and helping you to be grounded in incarnation.
- Energy and protection can flow up this root to keep you energized and safe.

You can extend this exercise by allowing the roots to pass up through your feet, up your legs and into your hips. At your hips the roots move across to meet in the base chakra, and from there to the sacral and the dantien. The energy that flows up from the centre of the Earth can be stored in the dantien.

> *Note:* Whenever you are in an area of seriously disturbed earth energy, protect your Earth Star chakra by visualizing a large Smoky Quartz or Smoky Elestial Quartz all around it. The root will still be able to pass down to the centre of the earth to bring powerful energy to support you, and the crystal will help to transmute and stabilize the negative energy. Even a virtual crystal can work when visualized with intent, but placing an actual crystal here intensifies the effect.

See page 130 for a chakra layout to cleanse, heal and maintain balance.

Finding Your Prescription

Every body is different. Each person has their own unique vibration and bioenergetic field. So there is no 'one stone fits all' remedy – although Shungite probably comes closest for EMFs. Therefore you need to find the crystal or combination of crystals that works best for you. The best way to select your crystals and to identify where to place them is to dowse for them or choose them intuitively (see page 93). Most entries in this directory offer a choice of crystals to assist a particular condition or issue. While all the stones listed in the directory could potentially help you, selecting the right crystal is crucial if you are to obtain maximum benefit and the fastest relief or most effective harmonising and/or blocking. Some crystals have a much finer vibration than others, working from the etheric to adjust the physical, and some work at a physical level so you may need to use a series of crystals or combine them within a grid.

You may find that you are instinctively drawn to a particular stone, and it may be one that you already have in your collection. If so, try this one first.

You can also dowse when purchasing a healing crystal, either by allowing your fingers instinctively to pick the right stone from a number of stones – the one that 'sticks' to them – or using a pendulum or finger dowsing (see page 93). Dowsing is an excellent way to identify GS lines, and you can either use a pendulum for this purpose or finger, body or rod dowse (see page 95). Rods move inward and cross, or move outwards as they cross a ley or GS line, or enter an area of electromagnetic smog. All methods use the ability of your intuitive body-mind connection to tune into subtle vibrations and to influence your hands. A focused mind, trust in the process, carefully worded questions and a clear intent will support your dowsing and your healing.

Framing your question

Framing your question with precision is essential if you are to achieve the most beneficial result. Your questions need to be unambiguous and capable of a straight 'yes' or 'no' answer. They also need to be asked with serious intent. An irresponsible approach or a frivolous question is unlikely to reveal anything of lasting benefit and could actually do harm as crystals are powerful tools that pick up and amplify your thoughts – positive or negative. They should be treated with respect.

Take time to prepare yourself to ask the question. Sit quietly for a few moments, bringing your focus away from the outside world and quietening your mind. Word your question carefully. If, for instance, you ask: "Is this the right crystal for me?" The answer could well be "yes" but it may not refer to the condition you wish to relieve at that precise moment. It could indicate a crystal that would give you long-term benefit for an, as yet, unrecognised issue that exists at an emotional, mental or soul level. That crystal could well be of value to you in the long term, but it would not heal the immediate symptom or provide the protection you are seeking.

You need to be specific. If you are finger dowsing (see page 93), ask: "Is [name of crystal] the best and most appropriate crystal to treat my insomnia at this time?" If you are pendulum dowsing (see page 95), say: "Please show me the best and most appropriate crystal to treat my insomnia now." Asking, "Is my insomnia caused by GS or EMFs?" would reveal the underlying cause, which may need to be treated with different crystals. Finger or pendulum dowsing will also assist in selecting exactly the right place to position your crystal when creating an energetic net to absorb and transmute negative energies. You can also dowse to ascertain the best shape for the grid (see page 120).

Dowsing

There are several methods of dowsing so try them all until you find the one that works best for you and then practise to refine your technique. Dowsing for solutions works best in an energetically clear space, but dowsing can be used to find GS lines and areas of electromagnetic smog.

Finger Dowsing

Finger dowsing answers 'yes' and 'no' questions quickly and unambiguously, and can be done unobtrusively in situations where a pendulum might provoke unwanted attention. This method of dowsing works particularly well for people who are kinaesthetic, that is to say their body responds intuitively to subtle feelings, but anyone can learn to finger dowse.

To finger dowse

To finger dowse, hold the thumb and first finger of your right hand together (see illustration). Loop the thumb and finger of your left hand through to make a 'chain'. Ask your question clearly and unambiguously – you can speak it aloud or keep it within your mind. Now pull gently but firmly. If the chain breaks, the answer is usually 'no'. If it holds, the answer is usually 'yes' – but check by asking your name in case your response is reversed.

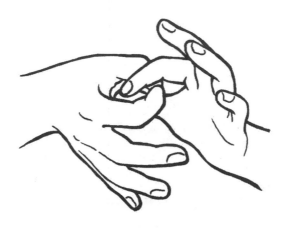

Finger dowsing

To rod dowse

You can use purpose-made dowsing rods, y-shaped hazel twigs or cut wire coat hangers into right-angled shapes. Hold the rods loosely in your hands, fingers curled inwards to make a holder, and slowly walk forwards across a room or site. Ask to be shown where the lines are. The rods will move or twitch when you reach the front edge and move back to straight when you pass out of it (see Finding GS lines and EMFs page 111).

Body dowsing

As bodies are extremely sensitive to changing vibrations you can use your hands or feet to dowse for GS lines or EMFs. If you are using your hands open your palm chakras (see page 87), extend them forwards with your palms turned up and facing out. Walk slowly and when you reach the line it will feel as though you are pushing against an energetic wall. Or, your feet may tingle if the line is beneficial, or your knees go weak and feel like you are walking through treacle if the line is harmful.

Pendulum dowsing

If you are familiar with pendulum dowsing, use the pendulum in your usual way. If you are not, this skill is easily learned. Crystal pendulums, especially Shungite or other EMF harmonisers or blockers are useful for this but wooden ones can also be used.

To pendulum dowse

To pendulum dowse, hold your pendulum between the thumb and forefinger of your most receptive hand with about a hand's length of chain hanging down to the pendulum – you will soon learn what is the right length for you. Wrap the remaining chain around your fingers so that it does not obstruct the dowsing.

You will need to ascertain which is a 'yes' and which a 'no' response. Some people find that the pendulum swings in one direction for 'yes' and at right angles to that axis for 'no', while others have a backwards and forwards swing for one reply, and a circular motion for the other. A 'wobble' of the pendulum can indicate a 'maybe' or that it is not appropriate to dowse at that time, or that the wrong question is being asked. In which case, ask if it is appropriate and, if the answer is 'yes', check that you are framing the question in the correct way. If the pendulum stops completely it is usually inappropriate to ask at that time.

You can ascertain your particular pendulum response by holding the pendulum over your knee and asking: "Is my name [correct name]?" The direction that the pendulum swings will indicate 'yes'. Check by asking: "Is my name [incorrect name]?" to establish 'no'. Or, you can programme in 'yes' and 'no' by swinging the pendulum in a particular direction a few times, saying as you do: "This is yes," and swinging it in a different direction to programme in 'no'.

To ascertain the best crystal for you

To ascertain which crystal will be most beneficial for you or for your purpose, hold the pendulum in your most receptive hand. Put the forefinger of your other hand on the condition or issue in the Directory. Slowly run your finger along the list of possible crystals, noting whether you get a 'yes' or 'no' response. Check the whole list to see which 'yes' response is strongest as there may well be two or three that would be appropriate, or you may need to use several crystals in combination. Another way to do this, if you have several of the crystals available, is to touch each crystal in turn, again noting the 'yes' or 'no' response – open your palm chakras before doing so (see page 87).

If you get a 'no' response when checking out a condition or site, open your palm chakras, touch each of the capital letters in turn, dowsing until you receive a 'yes', then run your finger down the conditions. This may well reveal something that underlies the apparent issue. If you get no response at all, it may be that you need to remove yourself from a geopathically stressed place, or that the question should be asked at another time.

Alternatively, open the palm chakras in your hands and allow your hands to simply find the right crystal, without thinking about it, which will feel tingly or may jump out of your hands as you pick it up.

How long should I use a crystal?

A pendulum can also be used to establish for how long a crystal should be left in place. This is particularly useful if you are placing the crystal at a site or over an organ or around your body or bed, but it can also be helpful if you are wearing a crystal and need to know whether or not to wear it at night – in which case you will get a 'yes' or 'no' answer to the question: "Should I remove this crystal at night?" To establish timing, use an arc on which you have marked five-minute or one-hour or one-day intervals (ask in advance whether the period should be checked in minutes, hours or days). Hold the hand with the pendulum over the centre of the arc and ask that the pendulum will go towards the correct period (see illustration). Most crystals that are an integral part of a grid will remain in place for long periods of time but you can dowse to see whether they need cleansing, moving or replacing.

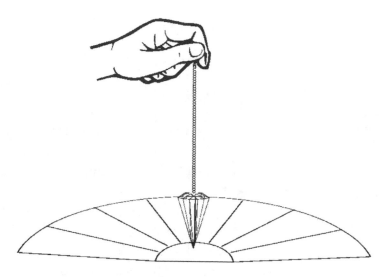

Dowsing over an Arc

Purifying and Focusing Your Crystals

Purifying Your Crystal

As crystals hold the energetic charge of everyone who comes into contact with them and rapidly absorb emanations from their surroundings as well as your personal energies they need regular purifying. This is particularly so when they are being used for healing, harmonising or blocking EMFs and GS. It is sensible to cleanse and re-energize a crystal every time it is used or at least weekly if in a grid. The method employed will depend on the type of crystal. Soft and friable crystals, for instance, and those that are attached to a base may be damaged by water, and soft stones such as Halite or Selenite will dissolve. These are best purified by a 'dry' process such as brown rice or sun or moonlight, but sturdier crystals benefit from being placed under running water or in the sea. Shieldite needs returning to the earth daily for fifteen minutes or so to keep it working at its optimum.

Remember, all crystals benefit from regular cleansing even those that may be described as never to need cleansing such as Shungite, which responds well to crystal clearing essences or immersing in brown rice. Re-energize in the light of the sun or with Clear2Light.

Methods:

Running water

Hold your crystals under a running tap, or pour bottled water over them, or place them in a stream or the ocean to draw off negative energy (use a bag to hold small crystals). You can also immerse appropriate crystals in a bowl of water into which a handful of sea salt or rock salt has been added. (Salt is best avoided if the crystal is layered or friable.). Dry the crystal carefully afterwards and place in the sun to re-energize or use a proprietary crystal essence.

Returning to the earth

You will need to dowse to establish the length of time a crystal needs to return to the earth in order to cleanse and recharge as the period will differ with each crystal. If you do not have a garden, a flowerpot filled with soil or sand can be used instead and is very handy for crystals that require a daily cleanse and regrounding. If you bury crystals to cleanse them, remember to mark the spot.

Rice or salt

Brown rice seems to have a special affinity with crystals that have been subjected to EMF pollution, rapidly drawing it off. Salt – and Halite – also works but can be damaging to layered or friable crystals). Place your crystal in a bowl of brown rice or salt (unless layered or friable) and leave overnight for the negative energies to be absorbed. (Brush salt off carefully and make sure that it has been removed from any niches or cracks in the crystal as otherwise it will absorb water in the future and could cause splintering.) Place the crystals in the sun to re-energize if appropriate or use a proprietary crystal essence. Compost or discard the rice, do not eat.

Smudging

Sage, sweetgrass or joss sticks are excellent for smudging as they quickly remove negative energies. Light the smudge stick and pass it over the crystal if it is large, or hold the crystal in your hand in the smoke if it is small. It is traditional to fan the smoke gently with a feather but this is not essential.

Visualizing light

Hold your crystal in your hands and visualize a column of bright white light coming down and covering the crystal, absorbing anything negative it may have picked up and restoring the pure energy once more. If you find visualization difficult, you can use the light of a candle. Crystals also respond well to being placed in sun or moonlight to cleanse and recharge.

Crystal clearing essences

A number of crystal clearing essences are available from

flower essence suppliers, crystal shops and the Internet (see Resources). Personally I never move far without Clear2Light, a crystal and space clearing essence. You can either drop the essence directly on to the crystal, gently rubbing it over the crystal with your finger, or put a few drops into clean spring water in an atomiser or spray bottle and gently mist the crystal.

If a grid has been buried, you can sprinkle a few drops of the essence into the general area and ask that it will cleanse and re-energize all the crystals in the grid. Petaltone Z14 is particularly helpful for grids as it clears fourteen layers of the etheric as well as the physical. Place a drop in the centre and invoke Archangel Michael to assist in clearing the area. Z14 can also be placed on a crystal such as Quartz or Selenite and left in situ to clear an area or to keep a crystal grid purified.

Re-Energizing Your Crystal

Crystals can be placed on a Quartz cluster or on a large Carnelian to re-energize them. Or, you can use a proprietary crystal recharger (Petaltone and the Crystal Balance Company make excellent ones, see Resources) but the light of the sun is an excellent natural energizer. Red and yellow crystals particularly enjoy being placed in the sun, and white and pale-coloured crystals respond well to the moon. (Be aware that sunlight focused through a crystal can be a fire hazard and delicate crystals will lose their colour quickly if left exposed to light.) Some brown crystals, such as Smoky Quartz, respond to being placed on or in the earth to recharge. If you bury a crystal, remember to mark its position clearly.

Focusing and Activating Your Crystal

Crystals work best when their energy is harnessed and focused with intent towards the task at hand as this activates them. By taking the time to attune a crystal to your own unique frequency, you enhance its vibratory effect and amplify its healing power. Once your crystal has been purified and re-energized, sit quietly holding the crystal in your hands for a few minutes until you feel in tune with it. Picture it surrounded by light and love. State that the crystal is dedicated to the highest good of all who use it. Then state very clearly your intention for the crystal – that it will heal or protect you, for instance, or that it will transmute negative energy. If it is intended for a specific purpose such as healing a particular condition, harmonising or blocking GS or EMFs, state that also. Repeat the intention several times to anchor it into the crystal.

Crystal Essences

Crystal essences are an excellent way to use the healing power of crystals, and several crystals can be combined provided you dowse to check compatibility. The essence can be gently rubbed on the skin or sprayed into a room. Essences intended for adult use are usually added to a glass of water and sipped, or taken from a dropper bottle, or sprayed around the aura or environment. Crystal essences are made by transferring the subtle energies and minute concentrations of the mineral constituents of the crystal into water, which then stores the vibrations and transfers them to the physical or subtle bodies in exactly the same way that a homoeopathic essence works. The essence is bottled and a preservative – brandy, vodka or cider vinegar – added. If the essence is to be taken by those for whom alcohol is inappropriate, cider vinegar can be used as a preservative or the essence rubbed on the skin. (See Resources for purpose-made highly effective essences.)

Caution: Some stones contain trace minerals bound up within them that are toxic (see the list in Contraindications) and essences from these stones need to be made by an indirect method that transfers the vibrations (see page 182). If in doubt, make the essence by the indirect method, which is also suitable for fragile or layered stones. Always wash your hands after handling one of these stones, and use in a tumbled version wherever possible.

Making a Crystal Essence

You will need the appropriate crystal, which has been cleansed and purified (see pages 99–102), one or two clean glass bowls, spring water and a suitable bottle in which to keep the essence (coloured glass is preferable to clear as it preserves the vibrations better). Essences can be made by the direct or indirect method. The indirect method is suitable for friable, layered or clustered crystals as well as those that may have a degree of toxicity. Spring water should be used rather than tap water that has chlorine, fluoride and aluminium added to it. Water from a spring with healing properties is particularly effective.

Direct method

Place enough spring water in a glass bowl to just cover the crystal. Stand the bowl in sunlight for several hours. (If the bowl is left outside, cover with a glass lid or cling film to prevent insects falling into it.) If appropriate, the bowl can also be left overnight in moonlight.

Indirect method

If the crystal is toxic or fragile (see Contraindications page 182) place the crystal in a small glass bowl and stand the bowl within a large bowl that has sufficient spring water to raise the level above the crystal in the inner bowl. Stand the bowl in sunlight for several hours. (If the bowl is left outside, cover with a glass lid or cling film.) If appropriate, the bowl can also be left overnight in moonlight.

Bottling and preserving

If the essence is not to be used within a day or two, top up with two-thirds brandy, vodka, white rum or cider vinegar to one-third essence, otherwise the essence will become musty. This makes a 'mother tincture' that can be further diluted. To make a small dosage bottle, add seven drops of the mother essence to a dosage bottle containing two-thirds brandy and one-third water. If a spray bottle is being made, add seven drops of mother essence to pure water if using immediately. For prolonged use, vodka or white rum makes a useful preservative as it has no smell.

Using a crystal essence

For short-term use, an essence can be sipped every few minutes or rubbed on the affected part. Hold the water in your mouth for a few moments. If a dropper bottle has been made, drop seven drops under your tongue at regular intervals until the symptoms or condition ceases. Essences can also be applied to the skin, either at the wrist or over the site of a problem, or added to bath water.

If a spray bottle is made, spray all around the aura or around the room. This is particularly effective for clearing negative energies, especially from the crystals themselves, or from a sickroom or an electromagnetically or emotionally stressed place.

Making Shungite water

To become biologically active, water needs to have Shungite immersed in it for at least 48 hours. However, once the first batch is made, you can simply refill the filter jug every time you use some of the water so that it is constantly replenished. Wash the jug and the bag of Shungite at least once a week depending on how much water you have used (you can store the activated water and return it to the jug). Place the Shungite in the sun for a few hours to recharge or use a proprietary crystal recharging essence. I find raw Shungite more effective than the silvery tumbles, but, no matter how often the non-vitreous type of Shungite has been washed, it does tend to leave a very fine suspension of black particles in the water. I have drunk this for several years now without any ill effects and, indeed, I believe it to have contributed greatly to my overall well-being.

Making the water:
You will need:
2-litre filter jug

Fine mesh 2″ bag of raw Shungite (10–100gm)

Place the mesh bag of Shungite in the base of the filter jug (if using tap water you can also use a commercial filter if the jug is provided with one). Pour water into the jug until it is full. Stand it aside for 48 hours. Then top up the water each time it is used. Cleanse the Shungite frequently under running water and re-energize.

Using your crystals

Crystals can be used either to mitigate the effects of GS and EMFs, to harmonise them so that your body can cope, or to deflect or block them altogether. Many of the directory entries indicate a chakra link through which a condition can be healed, or you can dowse for or intuit this (see page 93 and *Crystal Prescriptions 1 and 2* for further information on the physiology of the chakras). Most crystals can be placed over clothing on the chakra, or over organs or the site of dis-ease and left in place for 15–20 minutes or so. They can also be placed around the body, out in your aura or in your space or the environment to create energetic grids. If you are combating GS, grids can be buried directly into the ground (choose dark, robust stones such as Black Tourmaline or Smoky Quartz and mark the spot so that the crystals can be cleansed regularly) or stones can be inserted into the ground as stone needles. Crystals can also be taped in place, or worn for much longer periods for healing or prevention; or they can be kept in a pocket, or permanently placed around your bed or a room, or against a source of detrimental EMFs.

If your crystal has a point, place it point towards yourself, or point down if placed on your body, to draw in healing or re-energizing properties into your body. Place it point out, or point down below your feet to draw off toxic residues or emotional debris. If you are protecting your home, place the crystals point out to deflect or redirect negative energy and to harmonise the space. If you are drawing in beneficial energies, place the crystals point in. When you have placed the stones, close your eyes and breathe gently and evenly, and allow yourself to relax and feel the energy of the crystal radiating out through your whole being or your environment. Hold the intention that the stones will work for you.

You can also apply crystal essences (see pages 106–107). These essences convey crystal vibes to the body or the environment at a subtle level, repatterning your cells to their optimum.

Healing challenge

Occasionally a crystal, especially when used for EMF or GS clearing, will trigger a 'healing challenge' when the symptoms appear to get worse rather than better and flu-like symptoms may occur. This is an indication of physical, emotional or mental toxins leaving the body, or your environment, and is all part of the body holistically healing itself. It occurs particularly in stress-related or chronic conditions. It can be soothed and facilitated by crystals such as Smoky Elestial Quartz, Eye of the Storm, Spirit Quartz or Quantum Quattro and by drinking plenty of water (Shungite-infused water is ideal). If a healing challenge occurs use these stones for a few days until the symptoms dissipate and then return to the crystals you were using – having dowsed or intuited if they are still appropriate.

Finding GS Lines and Electromagnetic Smog

You can employ a professional dowser or anti-GS practitioner to check out your house, workspace or environment for GS lines, but it is very easy to find these for yourself. You can either work over a plan of the space or on a map, as many professionals do, or in the space itself. Rods, pendulums or body dowsing are all suitable methods for identifying the lines. You will need to check out how wide a line is, as well as the direction it moves in and any other lines that may cross it. A crossing point benefits from a large Smoky Quartz or other harmonising or blocking crystal, and lines can be gridded – dowse for where to place crystals. Rooms often have several lines criss-crossing them and lines may bend. It's helpful to make a sketch as you work to keep track of them (see below). Dowsing can also assist in ascertaining exactly how far EMFs radiate from electrical equipment.

Remember that your car may well be subject to geopathic stress if it regularly stands on a stress line, or to EMFs, so check that out and place crystals appropriately within it.

To find a GS line in a room or out in the environment

If you are using a pendulum, ask it to show you the GS and hold it in front of you as you very slowly move in a grid-like pattern up and then across and down until you have covered the whole area. Mark the points where the pendulum responds – remembering that lines are not always straight. Check that there are no other lines in the room by continuing the grid pattern, and working across the room in the other direction. You will probably find several.

If you are using rods, repeat the action above, watching for a response from the rods.

If you are finger dowsing, keep pulling your fingers until they hold together to indicate you have reached the line and open again when you have passed it.

If you are body dowsing, open your palm chakras and walk forwards, palms out. Or walk slowly placing your attention on your feet. Notice if your palms or feet tingle or go cold at certain spots or if it feels as though you are pushing against a wall of energy. Walk the same grid pattern so that you cover the whole room.

Note: If you are dowsing a bedroom and find GS lines, try to move your bed into a GS free space and neutralise the lines with crystals. You may also need to move your mobile phone out of your bedroom as this is a major cause of EMF smog and disturbed sleep.

To neutralise the lines

Place appropriate crystals at each end of the line where it enters a space and within that space wherever your dowsing suggests would be beneficial, especially at crossing points or where the lines enter a building and around a bed.

In the example plan shown below, there is a particularly strong line from a mobile phone mast (cell tower) passing through a bedroom (line A-B) and two other lines running from electricity poles and ground water cross it. Large Smoky Quartz crystals were placed at the crossing points on the ground outside to deflect, harmonise and redirect the energies and replace them with beneficial vibes, together with large external crystals on the major line and other minor lines towards

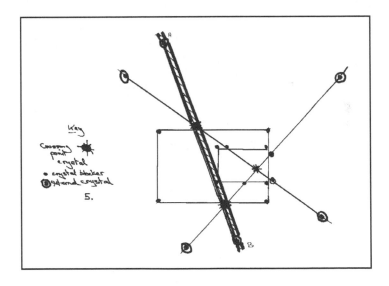

the property's boundary. A large Smoky Elestial Quartz was placed under the bed at the crossing point of the minor lines to transmute the effects. Black Tourmaline blockers were placed around the bed, on the lines and at the four corners of the room as the bed could not be repositioned. As the effect of the crystals kicked in, the placements were redowsed and crystals slowly removed until the optimum number was reached.

To find a GS line on a map or plan

If you are using a pendulum, ask it to show you the GS and hold it over the map or plan slowly moving it in a grid-like pattern up and then across and down until you have covered the whole plan or area. Mark the points where the pendulum responds (remember that lines are not always straight) and then join them up so that you see the line marked on the plan.

If you are using rods, repeat the action above, watching for a response from the rods.

If you are finger dowsing, keep pulling your fingers until they hold together to indicate you have reached the line and open again when you have passed it.

If you are body dowsing, open your palm chakras and use a forefinger to trace the grid-like pattern and notice if your finger tingles or goes cold at certain spots.

To neutralise the lines

Place your plan where it will not be disturbed, then place appropriate crystals at each end of the line or wherever your dowsing suggests would be beneficial. The map and the site will entrain. If possible also place crystals in the actual site.

What's in a Shape?

Crystals are found in many forms, some natural, others shaped. The shape of a crystal can affect how its energy flows:

A point directs energy in the direction it faces so remember to face all the points in a layout in the same direction to smooth the energy flow. Similarly, facing a pointed crystal towards the source of EMFs can deflect the energy away from you and break up the flow. Or it can assist in harmonising the energy field with your personal field.

In a **cluster** small, or large, crystals radiate out from a base pulsing energy out to the surrounding environment, and clusters can also absorb and harmonise detrimental energy.

The roundedness of **spheres and eggs** resonates particularly well with the human bioenergetic field and helps energy to flow gently in all directions. They are useful placed by or under a bed, or where stagnant energy needs to move smoothly, or fast energy be slowed down.

Pyramids assist with balancing and harmonising energy fields or fault lines but the shape is 'strong' and may be best kept out of the bedroom to ensure a good night's sleep. Place a pyramid at each end of a geopathic stress line as it passes through a house to negate the detrimental effect.

Cubes are particularly useful placed on or around computers or TVs to transmute the energy. They are extremely stabilizing and grounding.

A geode is hollow with many crystals pointing inwards. Useful for protection and conservation of energy, geodes hold and amplify energy diffusing the effect slowly, and softening the energy.

Raw **chunks** of suitable stone stabilize and transmute energy, and are best placed at the corners of a house or alongside the front door to protect the home environment.

Tumbled stones are particularly useful for wearing to protect your energy, but they can also be placed in grids.

Raw or polished?

In my experience, raw stones can be extremely useful. They may not be pretty but they soak up negative energies exceptionally well, acting like a sponge. Polished stones radiate beneficial vibes. Polished or faceted may be more comfortable to wear but raw stones, while not as attractive, can be worn with great effect.

Borrowing virtue

Your crystals don't need to be massive to work and there is a simple technique which boosts the power of smaller ones. Place them on a large version of the same crystal and hold the intention that the energies will entrain to work together at their most powerful when the smaller crystal is positioned in the landscape or used for healing (see pages 119-131).

Healing Layouts

Crystals are very effective when laid out in grids, simple patterns that encompass, purify, generate and amplify energy. They can be used for personal or space healing or environmental clearing, and to correct geopathic stress. The grids will need regular cleaning. If used for environmental clearing outdoors, the crystals can be buried in the ground but be aware that crystals such as Selenite will dissolve, and layered or clustered crystals may fragment. It is better to use tough stones like Black Tourmaline, Smoky Quartz or Preseli Bluestone which will, to some extent, be self-cleaning – unless of course you want to use the cleansing properties of Halite or Hanksite, which will detoxify negative energy as they dissolve (replace this type of grid if necessary after a few months). Remember to mark the spot, however, so that you can cleanse the crystals when necessary – this can be done by pouring water with a proprietary crystal cleanser and recharger into the ground over the crystals, or sprinkle a drop or two of the essence into the centre (Z14 is excellent for this). You can place a crystal near to a source of pollution or, to keep a whole house energetically clear, place a Chlorite Quartz point down in the

lavatory cistern so that each time it is flushed negative
energy is cleared away.

Chakra layout

A very simple but effective layout for healing personal
dis-ease and bringing your body back into balance is to
place a cleansed and activated crystal over each of your
chakras – you can dowse or intuit which crystals are
suitable and which of the minor chakras should be
included (see diagram on page 81).

- Begin with your feet and lay an appropriate
  grounding stone below and between them.
- Then place the crystals over the chakras moving up
  your body and slowly lying down as you do so.
- Finally place one or more at the top of your head.
- Relax and lie still for about fifteen minutes feeling
  the energy of the crystals harmonising your body
  and auric field.
- Then gather up the crystals in the reverse order
  that you laid them down – i.e. beginning with the
  one(s) above your head.
- When you reach the crystal beneath your feet,
  place your hands on it for a few moments to
  ground your energy before getting up.

Crystal grids

Placing crystals in a geometric pattern around your body,
bed, home or environment creates an energetic net that

purifies, heals and rejuvenates your energies, bringing in harmony and well-being and shielding where appropriate. Placing them around your space in a grid cleanses and protects the environment. Place the crystals at the points of the geometric figures. You can insert them into the ground if appropriate. Placing the crystals on a photograph or map is also effective. After you have laid out the crystal grid, join up the points with a wand or long-point crystal such as a Lemurian Seed.

Dowse or ask for the highest possible guidance as to which crystals are suitable for your particular layout as the circumstances change with each layout *and the person placing them*. Do ensure that your own energies have been cleansed and are at their optimum before commencing. Keep your thoughts and emotions calm, bring only positive energy to the task. Remember to prepare your crystals carefully. Putting 'uncleansed' crystals or fearful thoughts into a layout may not only throw the layout off balance but also negate the intended effect. The same goes for negative statements made near a layout. It picks up and amplifies the negativity. Avoid idle chatter or toxic thoughts, and remain positive.

Square (or rectangle)

Crystals:
4 cleansed and activated crystals

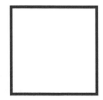

Lay one crystal at each corner of a room or around a building, your bed or in the environment to neutralise an EMF or GS source. Join the points with a long point crystal or the power of your mind.

Triangulation

Crystals:
3 cleansed and activated crystals

Lay one crystal above your head or centrally along a wall. Position the other two at the points of the triangle below your feet or in each corner of the room. Connect the points with a wand to strengthen the grid. Protective triangulation neutralises negative energy and brings in positive well-being. This layout is particularly helpful placed around your bed.

Zigzag

Crystals:
8 or more cleansed and activated crystals

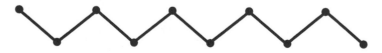

This layout is particularly helpful for sick building syndrome (SBS), or to counteract environmental pollution. It also pulls energy up from the Earth to ground you, or draws down spiritual energy from the higher crown chakras. You can adjust the number of stones to fit the space. Lay in a zigzag pattern so that the crystals touch the walls on either side, or are placed on either side of your body. It can be helpful to alternate high vibration crystals such as Selenite with cleansing stones such as Black Tourmaline or Smoky Quartz. Remember to cleanse the crystals regularly.

Star of David

Crystals:
6 cleansed and activated crystals

A traditional protection layout, placing the first triangle point down and joining the points, locks in negative energies for transmutation. Lay the second triangle over the top and join the points to draw in beneficial energy. The Star of David can also be used to draw in abundance and beneficial energies, in which case lay the first triangle point up to draw in the energies and place the second triangle point down to lock them in place.

Figure of eight

Crystals:
3 cleansed and activated high vibration stones such as new generation Quartzes

3 cleansed and activated grounding stones (see page 201)
1 synthesizing stone such as Elestial Quartz, Polychrome
Jasper or Shiva Lingam

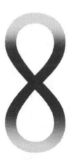

Drawing high vibration energy down into the body or
the environment, the figure of eight layout synthesises it
with earth energy drawn up from the feet to create
equilibrium and ground the raised vibrations. It creates
core energy solidity that enables riding out energetic
changes.

- Place the joining stone just below your navel or at
  the centre of the layout.
- Place a high vibration crystal at shoulder level, or
  halfway up the upper side, one at the top of your
  head or of the layout, and one halfway down the
  next side.
- Place a grounding stone level with your knees or
  halfway down the lower portion.
- Then one beneath your feet or at the base of the
  layout.

- Place the final one level with the one at your knees.
- Remember to complete the circuit back to the first stone placed.

This layout is also useful placed over a map to harmonise disruptive or disrupted earth energies.

Sunburst layout

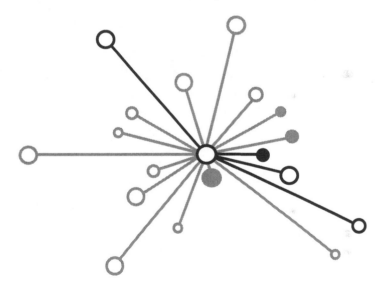

Sunburst

A radiating starburst energizes a whole area and is particularly useful for earth cleansing or harmonising via a map but it can also be laid out on the ground or buried within it if it is to be a permanent feature (remember to mark the spot so that you can cleanse the crystals). Although it is usual to start in the centre and work out, it can be helpful to dowse for the placements as a central alignment may need to be set out first or crystals placed to draw energy in. Crystals may be laid along each arm or at its end. The layout can always be adjusted to fine-tune the energies. This layout does not need joining with a wand to complete a circuit as the intention is to radiate the energy out as widely as possible.

Crystal placements

Large crystals can be placed next to the source of EMFs such as a TV, home hub, phone or computer or placed on a windowsill (dowse to ascertain the correct placement) or beneath where electricity cables enter your property. If the crystal has a point, face it in the direction you wish the energy to flow or towards where you need to divert it. A Chlorite Quartz point down in the lavatory cistern directs negative energy out of the building each time the lavatory is flushed, for instance. A Yellow Kunzite taped to your microwave helps to harmonise the energies so that they are no longer detrimental. And a laptop computer or tablet definitely needs a protective crystal especially if you are placing it in your lap. If there is an external EMF source near your house then point a large Smoky Quartz or Black Tourmaline outwards from the house to deflect, harmonise or neutralise the energy flow. Crystal spheres or polished, highly reflective crystals are particularly useful for slowing energy down or speeding it up smoothly as appropriate. They absorb stagnant and negative energy, and harmonise the flow of energy where this is creating GS. Placing crystals also works if there are high voltage electric pylons or cables, or cell phone masts near your home. Pointed crystals direct the energy flow in a specific direction and can deflect lines or harmonise them – and see page 225 for negative ionising crystals. Crystals don't have to be pretty and raw crystals often work just as well as polished ones, sometimes better if they are out in nature. Place crystals:

- Around your house, a single room, garden or a particular site to create a protective grid or to harmonise or deflect a GS line.
- In a specific area that is showing signs of GS deterioration.
- Next to electrical equipment in your home.
- On the base of a cordless phone or home hub.
- Stick one to a mobile phone, tablet or laptop.
- Around the base of a pylon or mobile phone mast – Black Tourmaline or Tourmalinated Quartz is ideal for this. Remember to do all masts in the area as the masts themselves can create an energy grid that boosts the detrimental effect.
- Either side of fault lines or in the centre of an earthquake area, or over tunnels or underground cables.
- Where there is chaotic energy in a house, such as a

small hallway with many doors leading off – place the sphere as close to the centre of the hall as possible against a wall so that the energy can flow smoothly around it and harmonise the space.

- In a long, narrow and dark hallway – place a polished crystal at the end of the hallway to reflect light back (Selenite or clear Quartz are excellent for this).
- Halfway down a set of rooms that open out of each other place a crystal to slow the rapid energy flow. (Smoky Elestial Quartz is ideal here.)
- At the top of the stairs if these lead immediately up from the front door so that energy reaches both floors equally.
- In a dark corner or dead end to avoid a build-up of stagnant energy and draw in light. (Selenite or clear Quartz is excellent for this.)
- If a road sweeps past carrying rushing energy with it, placing a sphere near or outside the front door or corner of the house calms the energy flow (Eye of the Storm is useful).
- When a house faces a road or stands on a corner so that dagger-like energy strikes it – place the crystal in a front window or next to the front door to divert the energy. (Eye of the Storm is useful as it calms the energy flow.)

CROSS ROADS

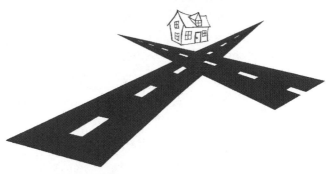

A house placed here would receive a dagger of fast moving energy from two directions where the roads intersect, which crystals placed outside the front of the house or just inside the front door could deflect. Energy could also rush past the house along the major road, and a crystal outside would slow it down and harmonise it if appropriate.

Outdoor layouts

If you are laying crystals out of doors, remember to choose robust stones that will not dissolve or shatter in frosty conditions. You can also add a central stone such as Halite or Selenite soaked in Petaltone Z14 or an environmental essence to keep the grid energetically clear, particularly useful if the grid is to be buried in the ground. The stone will eventually dissolve but that is part of the process.

1. Cleanse your stones and state your intention.
2. Open your palm chakras.

3. Select your spot by dowsing or use your intuition.
4. Lay the grid out roughly to begin with.
5. A long pole helps to establish that radiating lines are straight, or a ruler on a photograph can be used to check the alignment but you may have to allow for camera distortion.
6. Adjust the stones if necessary.
7. Join the lines of the grid if appropriate.
8. If the grid is to be left in place for a long period, it can be buried in the ground; but remember to mark the spot so that the crystals can be cleansed or include a central stone soaked in Z14.

Map layouts

Map layouts are particularly useful in large areas for neutralising GS from power sources, aerials and the like or at an area of disturbed earth energy. It can also be used for earth healing, or to support the beneficial energy of a sacred place and draw it towards you. Placing crystals on a map in a geometric pattern transfers the crystal energy to the area covered through entrainment. The layout does not have to be large to be effective and it can be left in place for long periods. As you lay out your crystals on a map, consciously feel that you are part of the whole, part of the living entity that is our planet. And feel your cosmic connection too, so that you draw in universal energy and unite the microcosm and macrocosm. Hold the intention that the Earth is healed and supported by the crystals.

Anchor stones

In the same way that a heel stone anchors the energy of a stone circle into the landscape, an outdoor layout or a map placement benefits from having an anchoring stone placed at some distance from it. Typical anchoring stones are Granite, Flint, Hematite, Quartz-rich rock or Milk (Opaque White) Quartz, and you can also use large Smoky Quartz or Smoky Elestial Quartz for this task.

Research findings

Regina Martino and Christel Barbier, a biogenergeticist and geobiologist, conducted studies as to how Shungite successfully supported the body's energetic system when a research subject was close to a cordless phone base or Wi-Fi field. Shungite placed on the phone's base reversed the detrimental effect of the radiated field. You can read their findings in Regina Martino's book *Shungite* (see Resources).

Case Histories

Sometimes all it takes to make a difference is a single crystal, at other times a combination is needed. These case histories have been selected to show how crystals have been used in a variety of situations. Adapt them to suit your own needs.

Sleepytime

A few years ago I was visiting friends in Mallorca. They had restored an ancient farmhouse in a beautiful garden and lived there for some years in peaceful tranquillity. Recently, however, the utilities company had built a high-voltage power line within yards of the property. It was so close you could hear the whine and hum of the power lines from inside the house. One of the owners could not sleep at all when in the house, and felt very frail and ill. His immune system was breaking down. His wife was feeling disorientated and strange, but had not yet developed physical symptoms. They had both taken to sleeping in an outbuilding some distance from the property and spent most of their time in the garden. They were about to sell the house. As I've already said, I am electrosensitive so it was a surprise that I could sleep within the property and felt at ease there. I was wearing a piece of Ajoite in Shattuckite, a rare combination which is very effective for neutralising EMF emissions. When I gave it to the owner, he had his first good night's sleep since the pylons had been installed. I, on the other hand, spent a dreadful night. We bought Black Tourmaline at a local crystal shop and placed them around the pylons and the house. However, the only thing to do was to sell as quickly as possible as no one who was electrosensitive should live that close to high voltage power lines. Indeed, I would say that no one at all should be expected to live that close.

Restoring harmony

A workshop participant spoke about the extreme difficulties she was encountering in her primary school classroom. The school adjoined an electricity substation, and construction work in the area was tunnelling deep into the ground. Stress and illness were rife in both teachers and pupils. Antisocial behaviour in the playground and aggression in the classroom had reached an all-time high. She was aware of a sense of constant background dis-ease. On the workshop the participants gathered together to assist. She dowsed for suitable stones to restore harmony and the group seeded them with loving intention. Fortunately her classroom had a high ledge around it and she placed raw Rose Quartz on it – having dowsed on a plan for the positions. She also kept a polished stone on her desk together with some tumbled stones for the children to hold. Largish pieces of Smoky Quartz were placed against the wall of the substation, and others were discreetly buried around the school's perimeter. She reported back that, almost instantaneously, harmony was restored to her classroom and from there to the school.

Rose Quartz also restored harmony in a Steiner community for special needs adults. A friend's son was moving to the community and she was extremely worried about the fact that the main electricity cable for the house came in above his window. He suffered badly from asthma and was electrosensitive. So we placed Rose Quartz and Black Tourmaline around his room. When he first moved in, one of the other occupants was extremely aggressive, complaining about the noise from football games her son was watching on television. Apparently this was nothing new; the occupant disliked change and was often aggressive – which might be explained by the building being geopathically and EMF stressed. But within a few days the two became good friends and everything calmed down. Coincidence? I don't think so. Rose Quartz had worked its magic once again.

Energy bombs

Geomancer Nicky Crocker kindly provided this case history to demonstrate how other people use crystals for anti-GS work.

It is with honour and privilege that I write this to be

included in Judy Hall's book. Judy's books especially *The Crystal Bible* have been instrumental in my learning and knowledge of the crystals I have used while dowsing and clearing people's homes and businesses for nearly 10 years. I have developed what I call an 'Energy Bomb', which is a compilation of minerals and crystals contained in a beautiful pyramid-shaped pot. These help to alleviate the effects of Geopathic Stress and Electromagnetic Smog: particularly Aventurine, Amazonite, Black Tourmaline, Smokey Quartz, Amethyst, Clear Quartz and more, depending on what people are suffering from. If there is more Electromagnetic Smog or stronger Geopathic Stress, then I will add more Black Tourmaline or Yellow Kunzite, Sodalite, and Malachite, Obsidian, Lepidolite, Brown Jasper, Agate, Turquoise, Larimar and Fluorite, depending on what I feel the customer needs.

My customers find these extremely calming, and have found they help alleviate sleep disorders, and create a calming effect in their homes. Depending on an individual's state of health, this may affect them in different ways, but everyone has stated they not only look good, but they also help them feel good as well.

Several years ago I dowsed a young lady's home in Sydney, and on arriving noticed two large cats. They are a good indicator for Geopathic Stress. It is interesting how many homes I find where the Geopathic Stress runs through parts which also coincide with where the cats like spending their time. At this client's apartment I found a strong line running through the lower part of her bed on both sides. The rest of her room was fine, however, it was not a large room and there was no other place we could realistically put her bed. I suggested using one of my 'Energy Bombs' after she told me the issues she was having with her legs. This included a knee injury that was not responding to physio treatment, and she was also suffering from twitchy legs during the night, which was diagnosed as 'Irritable Leg syndrome'.

Following further investigation, I decided the best place to situate the 'Energy Bomb' was directly under the bed, where her legs lay. She also informed me that her two cats loved sleeping exactly there on the lower part of the bed, which was interesting as no direct sunlight entered this room to reach the bed, and that they also slept there even if she was not in the room. There was another position in the house where the cats liked sleeping, which also had a Geopathic Stress line running through it, in addition to direct sunlight. However, the line where the bed was situated was their favourite. Cats are drawn to the warmth that the energy from Geopathic Stress creates and to them it feels good. Sadly, however, it is not so good for us, or dogs.

About a week later, the lady contacted me saying she had noticed the cats had stopped sleeping on her bed, and she had definitely noticed and enjoyed improved sleep. Also her irritable legs had dissipated.

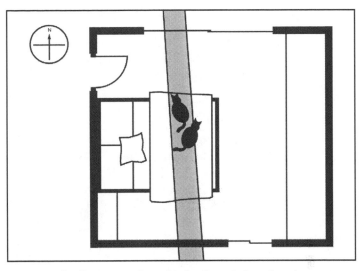

Note the line crossing the bed and the sleeping cats

Six months later she rang me again after noticing the cats had started sleeping on her bed again. I explained that the crystals probably just needed cleansing and recharging, so to put the 'energy bombs' out in the full sun or overnight in a full moon, and see what happened. She did this and the cats stopped sleeping on her bed again. I also explained that the 'Energy Bombs' filled with all these beautiful crystals would almost tell you when they need 'charging'. It's like when you walk into a room and you know you need to open a window to let in some fresh air.

While there is nothing wrong with a cat sleeping on a bed, we don't want that detrimental or negative energy where we are sleeping or spending extended periods of time in a stationary position (bed, couch, office, favourite chair etc.) to affect us healthwise. I have used the same 'Energy Bombs' filled with these amazing crystals for many years now and find they help alleviate, block, grid, stabilize, absorb, transform and protect against the negative effects of Geopathic Stress and Electromagnetic Smog, and have a definite calming effect on my customers. Some even like to take them on holiday with them.

– Nicky Crocker, 12 May 2014

And finally, to complete these case histories, an example from my book *Earth Blessings: Using Crystals for Personal Energy Clearing, Earth Healing and Environmental Enhancement*. New Zealand is on the 'ring of fire', a volcanic arc all around the Pacific Ocean. The constantly shifting plates create a vast amount of geopathic stress and in earth healing workshops we frequently work to calm this area by placing crystals on a map. After the Japanese earthquake and tsunami we placed Malachite on a map to soak up the radiation pollution together with Aragonite and Smoky Quartz to stabilize the energies. In the case below, circumstances were such that it was possible to position a crystal on the ground in Christchurch, which had been the epicentre of a series of devastating earthquakes leaving the area shocked and depleted, and keep it connected to a crystal anchor here in England.

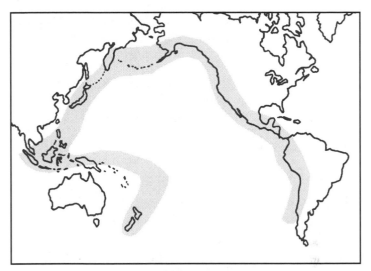

The Ring of Fire

Restoring energy in New Zealand

A friend who lived in Christchurch was experiencing constant violent aftershocks following a massive earthquake – there are over 15,000 earthquakes in New Zealand every year but this had been the biggest of them all. Her beautiful, peaceful home atmosphere had been wrecked by the energetic shock even though the house itself had withstood the quakes. Her own energy was shot to pieces too. There was clearly considerable geopathic and psychological stress in the area. Then came a second big quake. As she reported, "The whole community has lost so much over the past year and the level of fear has been terrible. Before yesterday the whole city precinct was just a skeleton of bones of buildings, now it will be a ghost city. The aftershocks are continuing around Christchurch on a lesser scale but the seismologists have warned us of the possibility of another big quake within the next 12 months so everyone remains nervous." The whole area needed calming and healing.

Page left New Zealand for a recuperative holiday and called in to see me in England. Fortunately I had just acquired two rather remarkable pieces of self-healed Quartz which had 'mountains' naturally etched into them. One was a smaller version of the other and we put them together so that the small one could 'borrow virtue' and work at its most powerful, the smaller one drawing on the energy of the bigger even when on the other side of the world. Page returned home and placed the crystal. This is her report:

Yesterday I settled the crystal next to the running stream of alpine waters at the front of my house – this is the place I saw when you handed it to me. The immediate surrounds are darkened by a natural dense canopy of graciously aged trees dressed by an undergrowth of softly entwined and interwoven foliage. Shafts of sunlight sparkle the water and if you sit quietly and withdraw from the external environment, you can hear voices from past times. As soon as I placed the crystal on the floor of leaves it immediately became incandescent and almost appeared to be radiating a living energy. The camera hasn't captured what I saw but you will be able to see beyond the imagery.

In the photograph (which is shown in *Earth Blessings*), the crystal glowed and the energy improved rapidly. I put the other one away quietly to do its work. I took it out a year later and my formerly lovely white stone had become murky and grey – a lesson to me to cleanse it more often. It quickly went out into a thunderstorm, was dipped a sacred well and placed in the sun for a recharge before taking up its work again.

If you live in an area that has been through any kind of earth-shock, a large clear or Smoky Quartz helps you to calm and restore the energies. Dowse or intuit its placement. Alternatively, you can bury large Aragonite crystals in the ground to stabilize the energy in your area or place them on a map.

Crystal Portraits

These are by no means all the crystals that assist with EMFs and GS (see Part II: A–Z Crystal Directory, and *The Crystal Bibles 1–3*) but they are some of the most useful.

Amazonite: cleans with a filtering action, absorbing EMFs and microwaves as well as mobile (cell) phone emanations. Place it on a computer or tape to a cell phone.

Amethyst: tunes the endocrine system and regulates metabolism. It wards off geopathic stress. Place by the bed to ameliorate insomnia.

Aragonite: an effective earth healer, Brown Aragonite grounds and stabilizes energy and transforms geopathic stress, unblocking ley lines. Place it on a map to heal energetic disturbance or to restore equilibrium. Centring physical energies and calming oversensitivity, it deepens your connection with the planet.

Aventurine: diffuses negative situations and absorbs electromagnetic smog. Tape it to a mobile (cell) phone.

Dowse to see which colour works best for you. Green Aventurine is an excellent spleen chakra stone, protecting you from energy vampires.

Black Tourmaline: a piezoelectric stone that generates a weak electric current, producing far infrared rays and converting moisture in the air to negative ions. Tourmaline neutralizes electromagnetic smog as well as many other environmental pollutants. Tape or glue to a cell phone, or place on a computer or other sources of electromagnetic smog. Grid to harmonise or block geopathic stress (see page 120) or wear constantly.

Flint: used from pre-history to protect and harmonise environmental energies and create a portal. It has the advantage of being free if you live in a Flint-rich environment and large pieces of Flint placed against the wall provide excellent protection from EMFs and redirect GS lines. Smaller pieces of Flint 'scrape down' and cleanse the aura, and repair breakages.

Fluorite: extremely effective against computer and electromagnetic stress and for reorganising your cognitive functions.

Halite or Hanksite: both these stones work well to purify an area. If you bury them in a grid they will dissolve and gently cleanse the surroundings. If you place them on a map they energetically cleanse the area.

You can cleanse your own energies with them by placing them in the bath or under the shower.

Hematite: this very useful grounding and strengthening stone improves your physical energy and helps attune you to the planet. It has a strong resonance with blood and helps to raise oxygen levels in your body.

Iron Pyrite: blocking negative energy and pollutants at all levels, Pyrite creates an excellent energy shield. Pyrite-rich Healer's Gold is particularly useful for creating a personal energetic interface that protects your energy field. It also helps to harmonise detrimental energy fields, adapting them so that your body can cope.

Jasper: is excellent at alleviating both geopathic and environmental stress, and harmonising or deflecting radiation. It draws toxins from the body and enhances energy levels. It is available in many varieties and colours. Dowse to see which one will work best for you. **Eye of the Storm (Judy's Jasper)** is particularly useful as it creates a calm centred space. Carry one with you at all times.

Kunzite: a protective stone that dispels negativity and geopathic stress. Yellow Kunzite deflects radiation and microwaves and can clear environmental smog by harmonising the energies to your own. Kunzite contains lithium and ameliorates dark moods; wear it constantly.

Lepidolite: mica based, this crystal is useful for clearing electromagnetic pollution. Place on computers or cell phones to clear the energy. It also enhances the generation of negative ions.

Obsidian: Apache Tear, Mahogany and Snowflake Obsidian can be extremely efficient in blocking geopathic stress or soaking up environmental pollution, but Black Obsidian can be fierce in its effect and create catharsis and energetic chaos. The other varieties are gentler as they harmonise the fields to your own energetic field.

Orgonite: this is not a natural crystal but it contains crystals of various types together with metal shards and other components. Orgonite neutralises and harmonises the harmful effects of EMF radiation when placed on devices. Orgonite also turns positive ions into negative, with a harmonising influence on the nervous system, moods, stress and overall health.

Quartz: composed of silica which is particularly effective for clearing electromagnetic smog and dispersing GS, Quartz generates beneficial piezoelectricity. Place it between you and the source of the pollution.

Rhodozite: although tiny, Rhodozite is an extremely powerful earth healer that enhances the effect of other crystals. Place it on maps and in layouts. As it rarely needs cleansing, it can be left to do its work. It can be placed to calm inclement conditions or to add vitality to the physical body or the planet as it enhances the flow of Qi (life energy) through the meridians.

Rose Quartz: a very gentle stone of infinite love and forgiveness that soothes aggression, Rose Quartz is nevertheless extremely efficient at harmonising or blocking GS and EMFs.

Shungite: the stone of choice for harmonising your energy body with other fields, and for blocking EMFs and GS and for creating good health. Shungite contains virtually all the minerals in the periodic table. It has phenomenal shielding power that arises from its unique formation. A rare carbon mineral it is composed of fullerenes, otherwise called 'Buckyballs' (spherical) or 'Buckytubes' (cylindrical). Fullerenes empower nanotechnology, being excellent geothermal and electro-magnetic conductors, and yet shield from EMF emissions. Wear Shungite or place on the source of electromagnetic frequency (EMF) emissions such as computers and cell phones to eliminate their detrimental effect on sensitive human energy systems (cleanse frequently). When doctors at the Ukrainian Academy of Medical Science carried out experimental protocols on patients who had undergone radiation therapy, the blood of the group drinking Shungite water returned to normal after two weeks whereas the control group took up to three to four months. There are two types of Shungite: the vitreous 'silvery-black' known as Elite that is very hard and shiny with silver and gold inclusions which is often found tumbled and looks silvery grey; and the greasier, blacker variety. The former can be placed as an anti-EMF or GS device and the latter used to make Shungite water.

Shungite transforms water into a biologically active life-enhancing substance, whilst at the same time removing harmful microorganisms and pollutants. Research has shown that Shungite absorbs that which is hazardous to health whether it be pesticides, free radicals, bacteria and the like, or EMF, microwave and other vibrational emissions. It boosts physical well-being and has a powerful effect on the immune system. Shungite-infused water is traditionally drunk two or three times a day to eliminate free radicals and pollutants, as an antibacterial and antiviral, and for prevention or lessening of the symptoms of the common cold and other diseases. A Shungite pyramid or sphere placed by the bed counteracts insomnia and headaches and eliminates the physiological effects of stress.[19]

No matter what you may read elsewhere, Shungite requires frequent cleansing and recharging as it rapidly absorbs negative vibes. (I use Petaltone Clear2Light or Temple Flame.)

Note: Shieldite and Fulgarite also contain EMF absorbing Buckyballs.

Smoky Quartz and Smoky Elestial Quartz: neutralize geopathic stress and transmute negative energy into beneficial vibes. Place one wherever there is GS or EMF overload.

Using This Directory

In the directory you will find an A–Z list of symptoms and common issues that may occur as a result of GS or EMFs with their appropriate healing crystals. Most entries have several crystals listed that would be beneficial, although a few have only one. There is a choice because everyone and every environment is subtly different and deeper causes may underlie a symptom. Crystals heal holistically – that is to say they work at a causal level on the whole person or the environment. What works for you may not necessarily work for your friend because you will have different causes for your dis-ease and you may well have different body types. Similarly, what is creating GS in one home may be very different to another that is affected close by which may be on a different line. Many of the entries also have a chakra or chakras associated with them. This means that the condition can be treated through putting appropriate stones on the chakra and leaving in place for 15–20 minutes or so. Or, the crystal can be placed in the environment or on a map – dowse for its precise position.

To identify the right crystal, check out your symptom,

condition or issue, and dowse or intuit which one(s) would be appropriate. If you have several symptoms, you may well find that one crystal is beneficial for all. This will be the crystal for you. It could be that you already own a crystal, having been instinctively drawn to it. But you may be left with a choice of several crystals, in which case turn to page 90 to learn how to identify the one that will be of greatest benefit to you, although many crystals work well in combination. Occasionally certain crystals are contraindicated and you will find these listed in the directory under Contraindications (page 182).

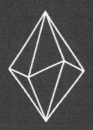

Part II

A-Z Crystal Directory

Crystals for combating EMF and GS

and healing associated disorders

- A -

Abdominal distension or colic: Aragonite (White), Carnelian, Snowflake Obsidian, Variscite. *Chakra:* sacral

ADHD (Attention deficit hyperactivity disorder): Amblygonite, Brandenberg Amethyst, Cumberlandite, Lepidocrosite, Stichtite, Tantalite, Tanzine Aura Quartz. *Chakra:* dantien. Place in pocket.

Adrenals: Aventurine, Axinite, Epidote, Eye of the Storm, Gaspeite, Jade, Nunderite, Picrolite, Richterite. *Chakra:* base, dantien, solar plexus

> **balancing:** Fire Opal, Rose Quartz, Yellow Labradorite
>
> **calming:** Cacoxenite, Eye of the Storm, Fire Opal, Green Calcite, Jamesonite, Kyanite, Rose Quartz, Richterite, Yellow Labradorite
>
> **overload:** Axinite, Eye of the Storm, Jade, Richterite

Adverse environmental factors: Aragonite, Amazonite, Black Tourmaline, Champagne Aura Quartz, Chlorite Quartz, Diamond, Ethiopian Opal, Fulgarite, Galena (wash hands after use, make essence by indirect method), Granite, Graphite, Heulandite, Khutnohorite, Marble, Natrolite, Petrified Wood, Pollucite, Preseli Bluestone, Orgonite, Scolecite, Shieldite, Shiva Lingam, Shungite, Smoky Amethyst, Smoky Elestial Quartz, Smoky Quartz, Stilbite, Thomsonite, Trummer Jasper. *Chakra:* earth star, dantien. Place crystal at four corners of house or site, on

---

Unless otherwise directed, place crystal in the environment or on a map, apply over an organ or site of symptom, place on an appropriate chakra, wear as jewellery, or bathe with or use as crystal essence.

computer etc.

Aggression, ameliorate: Amethyst, Blizzard Stone, Bloodstone, Carnelian, Fluorapatite, Pyrite in Magnesite, Rose Quartz, Ruby. *Chakra:* base, dantien

    use positively: Ruby Aura Quartz. *Chakra:* base

AIDS: Ametrine, Lapis Lazuli, Jadeite, Petalite, Quantum Quattro, Shungite, Zincite

Align:

    mind-body-spirit: Aurichalcite, Eye of the Storm, Golden Coracalcite, Green Ridge Quartz, Larvikite, Sillimanite. *Chakra:* alta major (base of skull) and dantien

    physical and subtle bodies: Alexandrite, Anandalite™, Aurichalcite, Empowerite, Fulgarite, Golden Coracalcite, Golden Healer, Green Ridge Quartz, Herderite, Lemurian Seed, Mount Shasta Opal, Nuummite, Paraiba Tourmaline, Schalenblende, Scheelite, Sillimanite, Thomsonite, Zincite. *Chakra:* alta major (base of skull), soma

    the chakras: Anandalite, Annabergite, Barite, Black Kyanite, Gaia Stone, Lepidocrosite, Lemurian Seed, Paraiba Tourmaline, Picrolite, Sichuan Quartz, Sillimanite, Sodalite, and see pages 171–178. *Chakra:* earth star to higher crown, dantien

Alzheimer's: Blue Obsidian, Eudialyte, Kunzite, Lepidolite, Purple Tourmaline, Rose Quartz, Rutilated Quartz, Shungite, Sodalite. *Chakra:* third eye. Place at base of skull.

Angina: Amethyst, Candle Quartz, Dioptase, Emerald, Magnesite, Rhodonite, Rose Quartz, Rhodochrosite. *Chakra:* heart, base

Antibacterial and antiviral: Amber, Anhydrite, Blue Euclase, Blue Tourmaline (Indicolite), Cathedral Quartz, Golden Healer Quartz, Green Calcite, Honey Opal, Iolite, Malachite (use as polished stone, make essence by indirect method), Proustite, Owhyee Blue Opal, Quantum Quattro, Que Sera, Shungite, Sulphur, Sulphur in Quartz, Trummer Jasper, Wonder Stone. Bathe in crystal essence, drink activated water or apply stone over site.

Anticarcinogenic: Champagne Aura Quartz, Klinoptilolith (wash hands after use, make essence by indirect method), Shungite and see Cancer page 167

Anti-inflammatory: Greenlandite, Shungite. *Chakra:* base. Or wear constantly, and see Inflammation page 209.

Antioxidant: Diaspore (Zultanite), Khutnohorite, Klinoptilolith (wash hands after use, make essence by indirect method), Piemontite, Reinerite, Shungite, Tantalite

Antiseptic: Amber, Amethyst, Blue Euclase, Calcite, Malachite (use as polished stone, make essence by indirect method), Quantum Quattro, Que Sera, Shungite. Bathe in crystal essence or apply stone.

Antisocial behaviour/aggression: Amethyst, Blizzard

Stone, Bloodstone, Carnelian, Eye of the Storm, Rose Quartz, Ruby, Sardonyx, Selenite, Sodalite. Place in environment.

Antispasmodic: Aragonite, Azurite, Diopside, Chrome Diopside, Magnesite

Antiviral: Amber, Cathedral Quartz, Fluorite, Honey Opal, Malachite (use as polished stone, make essence by indirect method), Quantum Quattro, Que Sera, Shaman Quartz, Shungite, Trummer Jasper. *Chakra:* higher heart

Anxiety: Amber, Aventurine, Chrysoprase, Emerald, Galaxyite, Green Calcite, Hematite, Khutnohorite, Kunzite, Labradorite, Lemurian Aquitane Calcite, Lemurian Gold Opal, Moonstone, Nzuri Moyo, Oceanite, Owyhee Blue Opal, Pyrite, Pyrite in Magnesite, Riebekite with Sugilite and Bustamite, Rose Quartz, Rutilated Quartz, Smithsonite, Scolecite, Strawberry Quartz, Tanzanite, Thunder Egg, Tiger's Eye, Tourmaline, Tremolite, Tugtupite. *Chakra:* earth star, base

Apoptosis (cell death and regeneration): Gabbro, Granite, Klinoptilolith (wash hands after use, make essence by indirect method). *Chakra:* dantien

Arteries:

   blocked: Larimar, Obsidian. *Chakra:* heart

   strengthen: Bloodstone, Stibnite

Arteriosclerosis: Aventurine, Magnesite

Arthritis: Amethyst, Apatite, Aztee, Azurite, Bastnasite, Blue Euclase, Blue Lace Agate, Brochantite, Calcite Fairy

Stone, Carnelian, Chalcanthite, Chalcopyrite, Chinese Red Quartz, Chrysocolla, Dianite, Fluorite, Garnet, Green Calcite, Hematite, Kinoite, Malachite (use as polished stone, make essence by indirect method), Nzuri Moyo, Obsidian (wear for short periods only), Paraiba Tourmaline, Plancheite, Prophecy Stone, Rhodonite, Rhodozite, Shungite, Wind Fossil Agate. Place over site and see Joints page 213.

Asthma: Amber, Amethyst, Ametrine, Apophyllite, Chrysoberyl, Dark-blue Sapphire, Iron Pyrite, Magnetite (Lodestone), Malachite (use as polished stone, make essence by indirect method), Morganite, Rhodochrosite, Rose Quartz, Tiger's Eye, Topaz, Vanadinite (wash hands after use, make essence by indirect method). *Chakra:* solar plexus, higher heart. Wear constantly over chest, use as crystal essence.

Atmospheric pollutants, remove: Black Tourmaline, Chlorite Quartz, Diamond, Elestial Quartz, Fulgarite, Graphite, Heulandite, Natrolite, Nuummite, Orgonite, Paraiba Tourmaline, Pollucite, Pyrite and Sphalerite, Quantum Quattro, Scolecite, Shaman Quartz, Shieldite, Shungite, Smoky Quartz, Sodalite, Stilbite, Thomsonite, Turquoise. *Chakra:* earth star. Or place in environment.

Aura: Anandalite™, Beryllonite, Quartz, Scolecite. Hold in front of solar plexus or sweep aura.

   align with physical body: Ajo Blue Calcite, Amber, Anandalite, Candle Quartz, Empowerite, Fulgarite,

Larvikite, Schalenblende, Scheelite, Scolecite, Sichuan Quartz, Sillimanite, Thomsonite. Hold over head or solar plexus.

blockages, remove: Ajo Quartz, Anandalite, Arfvedsonite, Beryllonite, Charoite, Fire and Ice Quartz, Flint, Fulgarite, Jasper, Prehnite with Epidote, Rainbow Mayanite, Rhodozite, Serpentine in Obsidian

cleansing: Amber, Amechlorite, Anandalite, Black Kyanite, Bloodstone, Citrine Spirit Quartz, Fire and Ice Quartz, Flint, Fulgarite, Green Jasper, Herkimer Diamond, Holly Agate, Keyiapo, Lepidocrosite, Mystic Topaz, Nuummite, Phlogopite, Pumice, Pyrite in Quartz, Pyrite and Sphalerite, Quartz, Rainbow Mayanite, Rutile, Smoky Quartz. 'Comb' aura thoroughly.

energize: Anandalite™, Gold in Quartz, Iolite, Quartz, Rainbow Mayanite, Sichuan Quartz, Triplite. *Chakra:* solar plexus

energy leakage, guard against: Eudialyte, Gaspeite, Healer's Gold, Labradorite, Pyrite in Quartz, Quartz with Mica, Spectrolite. *Chakra:* higher heart. Wear constantly.

heal: Anandalite, Keyiapo, Piemontite, Scolecite, Sichuan Quartz, Smoky Amethyst, Tugtupite

'holes'/breaks: Aegerine, Amethyst, Aqua Aura, Brookite, Chinese Red Quartz, Eye of the Storm, Flint,

Green Ridge Quartz, Green Tourmaline, Labradorite, Lemurian Seed, Quartz, Scolecite, Selenite. Place over site.

negativity, remove: Amber, Apache Tear, Black Jade, Fulgarite, Nuummite with Novaculite, Smoky Amethyst, Spectrolite, Tantalite. *Chakra:* solar plexus.

protect: Amber, Amethyst, Apache Tear, Brandenberg Amethyst, Diamond, Honey Phantom Calcite, Hackmanite, Labradorite, Mahogany Sheen Obsidian, Master Shamanite, Nunderite, Orgonite, Paraiba Tourmaline, Quartz, Shattuckite with Ajoite, Tantalite. *Chakra:* higher heart. Wear continuously.

seal: Actinolite, Andean Blue Opal, Brookite, Feather Pyrite, Fulgarite, Galaxyite, Honey Phantom Calcite, Healer's Gold, Labradorite, Lorenzenite (Ramsayite), Molybdenite in Quartz, Nunderite, Pyromorphite, Serpentine in Obsidian, Smoky Amethyst, Spectrolite, Tantalite, Thunder Egg, Valentinite and Stibnite, Xenotine

stabilize: Agate, Fulgarite, Granite, Labradorite, Mtrolite, Poppy Jasper. *Chakra:* earth star

strengthen: Ajo Blue Calcite, Anandalite, Brookite, Ethiopian Opal, Flint, Magnetite (Lodestone), Quartz Tantalite, Thunder Egg, Zircon

weakness, overcome: Brookite, Zircon

Autism: Cerussite, Charoite, Moldavite, Sugilite. *Chakra:* earth, base, solar plexus. Wear continuously or keep in

---

Unless otherwise directed, place crystal in the environment or on a map, apply over an organ or site of symptom, place on an appropriate chakra, wear as jewellery, or bathe with or use as crystal essence.

pocket.

Autoimmune diseases: Aquamarine, Bastnasite, Brandenberg Amethyst, Chinese Red Quartz, Diaspore, Gabbro, Granite, Golden Healer Quartz, Mookaite Jasper, Paraiba Tourmaline, Quantum Quattro, Que Sera, Rhodonite, Rosophia, Shungite, Tangerose, Titanite (Sphene), Winchite. *Chakra:* dantien, higher heart

Autonomic nervous system: Alexandrite, Anglesite Amazonite, Amber, Ametrine, Aventurine, Bloodstone, Charoite, Merlinite, Quantum Quattro, Que Sera, Sunstone, Tourmaline. *Chakra:* dantien

Back:

ache: Amber, Bloodstone, Blue Agate, Cathedral Quartz, Hematite, Iolite, Magnetite, Que Sera, Sapphire

disc elasticity: Aragonite

pain: Cathedral Quartz (over site of pain), Lapis Lazuli, Magnetite (Lodestone), Que Sera, Sapphire

Bacterial infections: Blue Tourmaline, Green Calcite, Malachite (use as polished stone, make essence by indirect method), Shungite. Bathe in crystal essence or place stone over site and see Antibacterial page 154.

Biological clock disturbances: Fluorapatite, Golden Healer Quartz, Kambaba Jasper, Menalite, Moonstone, Preseli Bluestone, Stromatolite. *Chakra:* dantien, higher heart, third eye or alta major (base of skull)

Biomagnetic field destabilized: Ajoite, Anandalite, Galena (wash hands after use, make essence by indirect method), Kyanite, Lepidolite, Magnetite, Orgonite, Preseli Bluestone, Quartz, Shungite, Sodalite, and see Aura page 156. *Chakra:* dantien, solar plexus

realign/strengthen: Angelinite, Astraline, Ethiopian Opal, Flint, Galena (wash hands after use, make essence by indirect method), Gold in Quartz, Golden Healer Quartz, Magnetite, Poldarvaarite, Pollucite, Preseli Bluestone, Quantum Quattro, Que Sera,

Unless otherwise directed, place crystal in the environment or on a map, apply over an organ or site of symptom, place on an appropriate chakra, wear as jewellery, or bathe with or use as crystal essence.

Shungite, Sodalite

Bipolar disorder: Bastnasite, Brucite, Charoite, Halite, Kunzite, Larimar, Lepidocrosite, Montebrasite, Peridot, Tantalite. *Chakra:* brow

Bladder: Amber, Bloodstone, Jade, Jasper, Orange Calcite, Prehnite, Topaz, Tourmaline, Vanadinite (wash hands after use, make essence by indirect method), Yellow Sapphire

Blood: Bloodstone, Cinnabar, Garnet, Sonora Sunrise, red stones. *Chakra:* heart, spleen

> **cells, red to white ratio:** Fuchsite, Tiger Iron
>
> **circulation:** Amethyst, Bloodstone, Carnelian, Galena (wash hands after use, make essence by indirect method), Garnet, Pink Tourmaline, Ruby, Seraphinite, Sodalite
>
> **cleanser:** Amethyst, Ametrine, Aquamarine, Bloodstone, Chlorite Quartz, Garnet, Hematite, Mookaite, Lapis Lazuli, Ruby, Tourmaline. *Chakra:* spleen
>
> **clots:** Amethyst, Bloodstone, Hematite
>
> **clots, dissolve:** Amethyst, Bloodstone, Hematite
>
> **clotting, improve:** Calcite, Red Chalcedony, Sapphire, Shattuckite
>
> **disorders:** Amethyst, Bloodstone, Blue Quartz, Chrysocolla, Cherry Opal, Fulgarite, Lapis Lazuli, Magnetite (Lodestone), Mookaite, Onyx, Prehnite, Sapphire

---

Unless otherwise directed, place crystal in the environment or on a map, apply over an organ or site of symptom, place on an appropriate chakra, wear as jewellery, or bathe with or use as crystal essence.

excessive clotting: Magnesite

faulty oxygenation: Amethyst, Carnelian, Chrysocolla, Kambaba Jasper, Stromatolite

flow in liver: Albite, Gaspeite, Mookaite, Variscite

poisoning: Carnelian, Quantum Quattro

purification: Angelite, Bloodstone, Pink Tourmaline, Sapphire

vessels: Fluorite, Fulgarite, Merlinite, Topaz

Blood pressure:

equalize: Aventurine, Charoite, Tourmaline. *Chakra:* heart, solar plexus

high: Amethyst, Bloodstone, Blue Chalcedony, Charoite, Chrysocolla, Chrysoprase, Dioptase, Emerald, Jade, Kyanite, Labradorite, Lapis Lazuli, Malachite (use as polished stone, make essence by indirect method), Rhodochrosite, Sodalite. *Chakra:* heart.

low: Carnelian, Red Calcite, Rhodochrosite, Ruby, Sodalite, Tourmaline. *Chakra:* heart

Blood sugar imbalances: Astraline, Chinese Chromium Quartz, Chrome Diopside, Citrine, Green Shaman Quartz, Huebnerite, Malacholla, Maw Sit Sit, Mtrolite, Muscovite, Orange Kyanite, Owyhee Blue Opal, Peridot, Pink Opal, Pink Sunstone, Rose Quartz, Serpentine in Obsidian, Shungite, Sodalite, Stichtite and Serpentine, Tugtupite, and see Diabetes page 189 and Pancreas page 230. *Chakra*: spleen, dantien, heart

---

Unless otherwise directed, place crystal in the environment or on a map, apply over an organ or site of symptom, place on an appropriate chakra, wear as jewellery, or bathe with or use as crystal essence.

Blueprint, etheric: Anandalite, Andescine Labradorite, Astraline, Black Kyanite, Beryllonite, Brandenberg Amethyst, Chlorite Quartz, Ethiopian Opal, Eye of the Storm, Fulgarite, Keyiapo, Khutnohorite, Lemurian Aquitane Calcite, Pollucite, Rhodozite, Ruby Lavender Quartz, Sanda Rosa Azeztulite, Scheelite, Seriphos Quartz, Tantalite. *Chakra:* soma

Body:

acceptance of: Candle Quartz, Eye of the Storm, Phenacite, Vanadinite (wash hands after use, make essence by indirect method). *Chakra:* earth, base, crown

discomfort at being in: Candle Quartz, Pearl Spa Dolomite, Quantum Quattro, Strontianite. *Chakra:* earth star, base, sacral, dantien

fluids, balance: Azeztulite with Morganite, Bastnasite, Hackmanite, Nunderite, Scheelite, Smoky Amethyst, Trigonic Quartz. *Chakra:* earth star, base, sacral

heat, excess: Brazilianite. *Chakra:* earth star, base, sacral

promote repair: Bixbite, Seraphinite, Tantalite, and see Cellular healing page 169. *Chakra:* earth star, base, sacral

rebalance: Shungite with Steatite, Victorite

strengthen: Blue Aragonite, Candle Quartz, Erythrite, Fiskenaesset, Peridot, Poppy Jasper, Ruby. *Chakra:*

Unless otherwise directed, place crystal in the environment or on a map, apply over an organ or site of symptom, place on an appropriate chakra, wear as jewellery, or bathe with or use as crystal essence.

earth star, base, sacral, dantien

work efficiently: Golden Healer Quartz, Phlogopite

Bone-marrow disorders: Cradle of Life, Goethite, Lapis Lazuli, Onyx, Violet-purple Fluorite

Brain: Amber, Amethyst, Beryl, Botswana Agate, Brandenberg Amethyst, Carnelian, Crystal Cap Amethyst, Epidote, Green Tourmaline, Kyanite, Labradorite, Magnesite, Nuummite, Prehnite with Epidote, Pyrite and Sphalerite, Royal Sapphire, Schalenblende, Sodalite, Staurolite, Trigonic Quartz, White Heulandite, Vera Cruz Amethyst. *Chakra:* third eye, soma, crown, alta major

balance left–right hemispheres: Crystal Cap Amethyst, Eudialyte, Hematite with Rutile, Hematite with Rutile Cumberlandite, Lilac Quartz, Rhodozite, Sodalite, Stromatolite, Sugilite, Trigonic Quartz. *Chakra:* soma

benign tumours: Scolecite

blood flow, improve: Iron Pyrite

chemistry: Barite, Stichtite

damage: Amphibole, Anthrophyllite, Brandenberg Amethyst, Galaxyite, Herderite

degeneration: Anthrophyllite, Sodalite

detox: Amechlorite, Chlorite Quartz, Eye of the Storm, Klinoptilolith (wash hands after use, make essence by indirect method), Lapis Lazuli, Larvikite, Nuummite, Rainbow Covellite, Rhodozite, Richterite, Ruby,

Shungite, Smoky Quartz with Aegerine, Sodalite, Thulite, Zircon

disorders: Brandenberg Amethyst, Chalcopyrite, Galaxyite, Holly Agate, Khutnohorite, Sapphire, Sodalite, Stilbite

dysfunction: Anthrophyllite, Blue Holly Agate, Cryolite, Cumberlandite, Sodalite

fatigue: Apricot Quartz, Pyrite in Quartz, Strawberry Lemurian, Turquoise

function: Cryolite, Phantom Calcite, Rhodozite

neural pathways: Anglesite, Celestobarite, Crystal Cap Amethyst, Feather Calcite, Feather Pyrite, Holly Agate, Larvikite, Phantom Calcite, Pyrite and Sphalerite, Schalenblende, Scolecite, Stichtite

stem: Blue Moonstone, Cradle of Life, Chrysotile, Chrysotile in Serpentine, Eye of the Storm, Kambaba Jasper, Schalenblende, Stromatolite

synapses: Azurite

tumour: Champagne Aura Quartz, Eilat Stone, Emerald, Klinoptilolith (wash hands after use, make essence by indirect method), Nuummite, Ouro Verde

Breathing disorders: Blue Aragonite, Blue Crackle Quartz, Hanksite, Morganite, Moss Agate, Riebekite with Sugilite and Bustamite, Tremolite, Vanadinite (wash hands after use, make essence by indirect method). *Chakra:* dantien, heart

Breathlessness: Amber, Amethyst, Apophyllite, Black

Onyx, Jet, Kambaba Jasper, Magnetite (Lodestone), Morganite, Moss Agate, Quantum Quattro, Que Sera, Stromatolite, Vanadinite (wash hands after use, make essence by indirect method). *Chakra:* higher heart, solar plexus, throat

Bronchitis: Amber, Black Onyx, Iron Pyrite, Jet, Kambaba Jasper, Pyrolusite, Rutilated Quartz, Shungite, Stromatolite

Unless otherwise directed, place crystal in the environment or on a map, apply over an organ or site of symptom, place on an appropriate chakra, wear as jewellery, or bathe with or use as crystal essence.

- C -

Cancer: Amethyst, Annabergite, Azeztulite, Azurite with Malachite (use as polished stone, make essence by indirect method), Bloodstone, Carnelian, Champagne Aura Quartz, Cobaltite, Covellite, Chalcopyrite, Cuprite with Chrysocolla, Diamond, Eilat Stone, Emerald, Fluorapatite, Fluorite, Gabbro, Gold in Quartz, Golden Healer Quartz, Green Ridge Quartz, Hematite, Heulandite, Kernite, Klinoptilolith (wash hands after use, make essence by indirect method), Lapis Lazuli, Lepidolite, Malachite (use as polished stone, make essence by indirect method), Malacholla, Magnetite (Lodestone) with Smoky Quartz, Melanite Garnet, Moonstone, Natrolite, Obsidian, Petalite, Pollucite, Quantum Quattro, Que Sera, Red Jasper, Reinerite, Rhodochrosite, Rhodozite, Sapphire, Scolecite, Selenite, Seraphinite, Shungite, Smoky Elestial Quartz, Smoky Quartz, Sodalite, Sonora Sunrise, Spinel, Stilbite, Sugilite, Thomsonite, Tourmaline, Ullmanite, Uvarovite, Xenotine and see Tumours page 247

> **support during:** Amethyst Spirit Quartz, Bixbite, Black Diopside, Brandenberg Amethyst, Cassiterite, Cathedral Quartz, Cobalto Calcite, Dendritic Chalcedony, Epidote, Eye of the Storm, Green Ridge Quartz, Hemimorphite, Icicle Calcite, Lemurian Jade, Paraiba Tourmaline, Quantum Quattro, Que Sera,

Reinerite, Rhodozite, Sonora Sunrise, Sugilite, Tremolite, Winchite

Candida: Carnelian, Zincite

Capillary degeneration: Dendritic Agate, Merlinite, Tektite

Car, neutralise EMFs: Black Tourmaline, Labradorite, Quartz, Shungite, Smoky Quartz. Keep in car.

Cardiovascular system: Kunzite, Peridot and see Heart, page 203

Carpal tunnel syndrome: Eye of the Storm, Fuchsite, Magnetite (Lodestone)

Cell phones: Amazonite, Black Tourmaline, Diamond, Orgonite, Shieldite, Shungite, Smoky Elestial Quartz, Smoky Quartz, Sodalite. Tape to phone.

Cells: Celestite, Dioptase, Garnet, Herkimer Diamond, Iron Pyrite, Staurolite, Yellow Kunzite

  detox: Chlorite Quartz, Eye of the Storm, Fulgarite, Klinoptilolith (wash hands after use, make essence by indirect method), Larvikite, Seraphinite, Shungite, Smoky Quartz with Aegerine

  energetic balance: Lemurian Gold Opal, Rainbow Covellite, Richterite, Sanda Rosa Azeztulite, Shungite. *Chakra:* dantien

  metabolism: Ammolite, Pyrite in Magnesite, Sardonyx, Tangerine Sun Aura Quartz

  production: Bixbite, Tantalite

  rejuvenation: Jasper, Rhodonite, Sodalite

Unless otherwise directed, place crystal in the environment or on a map, apply over an organ or site of symptom, place on an appropriate chakra, wear as jewellery, or bathe with or use as crystal essence.

repair: Bixbite, Glendonite, Rosophia

walls: Calcite Fairy Stone, Eye of the Storm, Feather Pyrite, Poppy Jasper, Titanite (Sphene). *Chakra:* dantien

Cellular:

blueprint: Ajoite, Ajo Quartz, Brandenberg Amethyst, Chlorite Quartz, Eye of the Storm, Fulgarite, Keyiapo, Khutnohorite, Rainbow Mayanite, Rhodozite, Ruby Lavender Quartz, Scheelite, Seriphos Quartz, Shattuckite, Yellow Kunzite. *Chakra:* higher heart, soma, alta major (base of skull)

detoxification: Chlorite Quartz, Eye of the Storm, Fulgarite, Kambaba Jasper, Larvikite, Rainbow Covellite, Richterite, Seraphinite, Shieldite, Shungite, Smoky Quartz with Aegerine, Stromatolite, Tantalite

disorders: Biotite, Celestite, Dioptase, Eye of the Storm, Garnet, Herkimer Diamond, Iron Pyrite, Pollucite, Pyrite in Magnesite, Reinerite, Rhodozite, Seraphinite, Shungite, Staurolite, Yellow Kunzite, Zoisite

disorganisation: Agnitite, Azotic Topaz, Biotite, Eklogite, Fulgarite, Golden Healer Quartz, Kambaba Jasper, Mangano Vesuvianite, Quantum Quattro, Que Sera, Reinerite, Rosophia, Sanda Rosa Azeztulite, Schalenblende, Shungite, Topaz

healing: Ajo Quartz, Brandenberg Amethyst, Crystal Cap Amethyst, Elestial Quartz, Eudialyte, Eye of the

Storm, Khutnohorite, Mangano Vesuvianite, Marialite, Nebula Stone, Pyrite in Magnesite, Rainbow Mayanite, Rainforest Jasper, Reinerite, Rhodozite, Rosophia, Schalenblende, Seraphinite, Tantalite, Titanite (Sphene), Zoisite

matrix: Eye of the Storm, Gold in Quartz

memory: Ajo Quartz, Ajoite, Andean Blue Opal, Azotic Topaz, Brandenberg Amethyst, Bustamite, Chrysotile, Datolite, Dumortierite, Eilat Stone, Elestial Quartz, Eye of the Storm, Heulandite, Leopardskin Jasper, Lepidocrosite, Nuummite, Rainbow Mayanite, Rhodozite, Sichuan Quartz, Smoky Quartz with Aegerine, Sodalite, Spirit Quartz, Valentinite and Stibnite. *Chakra:* dantien, alta major

micro level: Dendritic Agate, Fulgarite, Merlinite, Ruby Lavender Quartz, Seraphinite

processes: Eye of the Storm, Feather Pyrite

regeneration: Andean Blue Opal, Elestial Quartz, Eye of the Storm, Jasper, Lepidocrosite, Reinerite, Rhodonite, Rosophia, Seraphinite, Shungite, Sodalite, Tantalite, Zoisite

structure: Ajo Quartz, Ajoite, Bornite, Cradle of Life, Hausmanite, Indicolite Tourmaline, Lilac Quartz, Messina Quartz, Novaculite, Reinerite, Rhodozite, Selenite, Shattuckite, Shungite

wall reprogramming: Brandenberg Amethyst, Calcite Fairy Stone, Eye of the Storm, Feather Pyrite,

Unless otherwise directed, place crystal in the environment or on a map, apply over an organ or site of symptom, place on an appropriate chakra, wear as jewellery, or bathe with or use as crystal essence.

Fulgarite, Poppy Jasper, Seraphinite, Shattuckite, Titanite (Sphene). *Chakra:* dantien

Central nervous system, depleted or disturbed: Anandalite™, Alexandrite, Amethyst, Anglesite, Aventurine, Brandenberg Amethyst, Celestite, Dioptase, Fulgarite, Larvikite, Merlinite, Natrolite with Scolecite, Prehnite with Epidote, Rhodonite, Rose Quartz, Sodalite. *Chakra:* dantien. Wear continuously.

Centring: Bloodstone, Calcite, Celestobarite, Coral, Eye of the Storm, Flint, Fossilised Wood, Garnet, Hematite, Kunzite, Obsidian, Onyx, Peanut Wood, Quartz, Red Jasper, Ruby, Sardonyx, Tourmalinated Quartz

Chakras:

> **activate all:** Anandalite, Brookite, Fulgarite, Golden Healer Quartz, Green Ridge Quartz, Phlogopite, Rhodozite, Triplite, Victorite

> **activate higher crown:** Amphibole, Anandalite, Angel's Wing Calcite, Brookite, Diaspore (Zultanite), Glendonite, Golden Healer Quartz, Green Ridge Quartz, Lemurian Aquitane Calcite, Lepidocrosite, Merkabite Calcite™, Novaculite, Paraiba Tourmaline, Titanite (Sphene), Victorite. *Chakras:* soul star, stellar gateway. Place above head.

> **activate higher heart:** Ajo Blue Calcite, Macedonian Opal, Pink Lazurine, Pyroxmangite, Roselite, Ruby Lavender Quartz, Scolecite. *Chakra:* higher heart/thymus

align: Anandalite, Auralite 23, Brochantite, Citrine, Fulgarite, Golden Healer Quartz, Kyanite, Lemurian Seed, Montebrasite, Novaculite, Quartz, Rhodozite, Sillimanite

align with physical body: Amber, Anandalite, Candle Quartz, Celestial Quartz, Fulgarite, Keyiapo, Lemurian Jade, Lemurian Seed, Morion, Prasiolite, Preseli Bluestone, Rainbow Mayanite, Rhodozite, Seraphinite, Sichuan Quartz, Sillimanite, Smoky Herkimer Diamond, Thomsonite

Alta Major: Afghanite, African Jade, Anandalite, Andara Glass, Angelinite, Angel's Wing Calcite, Apatite, Auralite 23, Aurichalcite, Azeztulite, Blue Moonstone, Brandenberg Amethyst, Budd Stone (African Jade), Crystal Cap Amethyst, Diaspore (Zultanite), Ethiopian Opal, Eye of the Storm (Judy's Jasper), Fire and Ice Quartz, Fluorapatite, Garnet in Pyroxene, Graphic Smoky Quartz, Green Ridge Quartz, Diamond, Golden Healer, Golden Herkimer, Holly Agate, Hungarian Quartz, Petalite, Phenacite, Preseli Bluestone, Rainbow Covellite, Rainbow Mayanite, Red Agate, Red Amethyst, Rosophia. Place at base of skull.

balance: Anandalite, Auralite 23, Black Kyanite, Golden Healer Quartz, Lemurian Seed, Petalite, Seraphinite, Sichuan Quartz, Sunstone

base: Amber, Azurite, Bastnasite, Bloodstone, Candle

Unless otherwise directed, place crystal in the environment or on a map, apply over an organ or site of symptom, place on an appropriate chakra, wear as jewellery, or bathe with or use as crystal essence.

Quartz, Carnelian, Chinese Red Quartz, Chrysocolla, Cinnabar Jasper, Citrine, Clinohumite, Cuprite, Dragon Stone, Fire Agate, Fire Obsidian, Fulgarite, Gabbro, Garnet, Golden Topaz, Judy's Jasper, Kambaba Jasper, Keyiapo, Limonite, Pink Tourmaline, Poppy Jasper, Que Sera, Realgar and Orpiment, Red Calcite, Red Jasper, Serpentine in Obsidian, Shungite, Smoky Quartz, Sonora Sunrise, Stromatolite, Tangerose, Triplite. Place at perineum.

blockages: Ajo Quartz, Amechlorite, Anandalite (Aurora Quartz), Azurite, Bloodstone, Black Kyanite, Flint, Charoite, Chlorite Quartz, Fulgarite, Golden Healer Quartz, Green Ridge Quartz, Lemurian Seed, Picrolite, Prehnite with Epidote, Pyrite and Sphalerite, Quartz, Que Sera, Rainbow Mayanite, Rhodozite, Sanda Rosa Azeztulite

blown: Fire Agate

cleanse: Amethyst, Anandalite, Bloodstone, Calcite, Citrine, Enstatite and Diopside, Flint, Fulgarite, Golden Healer Quartz, Graphic Smoky Quartz (Zebra Stone), Orange Kyanite, Novaculite, Nuummite, Quartz, Rainbow Mayanite, Rhodozaz, Rhodozite

connect higher: Astraline, Angel's Wing Calcite, Rhodozaz, Rosophia, Titanite (Sphene)

crown: Afghanite, Amphibole Quartz, Angelite, Arfvedsonite, Citrine, Clear Tourmaline, Golden Beryl, Larimar, Lepidolite, Moldavite, Novaculite,

Quartz, Petalite, Phenacite, Purple Jasper, Purple Sapphire, Red Serpentine, Rosophia, Satyamani and Satyaloka Quartz, Selenite, Titanite (Sphene). Place on top of head.

dantien: Empowerite, Eye of the Storm, Golden Herkimer, Hematoid Calcite, Kambaba Jasper, Peanut Wood, Polychrome Jasper, Poppy Jasper, Red Amethyst, Rhodozite, Rose or Ruby Aura Quartz, Rosophia, Stromatolite

Earth Star: Agnitite™, Boji Stone, Brown Jasper, Celestobarite, Cuprite, Fire Agate, Flint, Galena (wash hands after use, make essence by indirect method), Graphic Smoky Quartz, Golden Herkimer, Hematite, Lemurian Jade, Limonite, Mahogany Obsidian, Proustite, Red Amethyst, Rhodonite, Rhodozite, Rosophia, Smoky Elestial Quartz, Smoky Quartz, Thunder Egg, Tourmaline. Place below feet.

energy leakage, prevent: Ajoite with Shattuckite, Black Tourmaline, Eudialyte, Gaspeite, Green Aventurine, Healer's Gold, Hematite, Labradorite, Pyrite in Quartz, Quartz Tantalite, Thunder Egg. *Chakra:* dantien, spleen, solar plexus

ground energies through: Aztee, Champagne Aura Quartz, Empowerite, Fulgarite, Keyiapo, Mohawkite (use as polished stone, make essence by indirect method), Peanut Wood, Polychrome Jasper, Red

---

Unless otherwise directed, place crystal in the environment or on a map, apply over an organ or site of symptom, place on an appropriate chakra, wear as jewellery, or bathe with or use as crystal essence.

Amethyst, Rhodozite, Schalenblende, Serpentine in Obsidian, Stromatolite, Thunder Egg. *Chakra:* earth star

heart: Aventurine, Cobalto Calcite, Danburite, Eudialyte, Gaia Stone, Green Siberian Quartz, Lilac Quartz, Pyroxmangite, Rhodozaz, Rose Quartz, Roselite, Rosophia, Ruby Lavender Quartz, Tugtupite. Place over heart.

heart seed: Ajo Blue Calcite, Brandenberg Amethyst, Danburite, Lemurian Calcite, Lilac Quartz, Macedonian Opal, Mangano Calcite, Pyroxmangite, Rhodozaz, Roselite, Rosophia, Ruby Lavender Quartz, Scolecite, Tugtupite. Place at base of breastbone.

higher crown: Anandalite, Apophyllite, Azeztulite, Celestite, Green Ridge Quartz, Kunzite, Muscovite, Petalite, Phenacite, Phenacite Kunzite, Selenite. *Chakras:* soul star, stellar gateway. Place above head.

higher heart/thymus: Ajo Blue Calcite, Danburite, Dioptase, Dream Quartz, Lazurine, Lilac Quartz, Macedonian Opal, Pink Petalite, Quantum Quattro, Pyroxmangite, Rhodozaz, Roselite, Rose Elestial Quartz, Rosophia, Ruby Lavender Quartz™, Tugtupite. Place over thymus.

holes, repair: Anandalite, Barite, Black Kyanite, Lemurian Seed, Novaculite, Rainbow Mayanite, Selenite

integrate higher: Anandalite, Fulgarite, Montebrasite, Petalite, Ruby Lavender Quartz™, Selenite, Titanite (Sphene)

palm: Flint, Spangolite. *Chakra:* throat, third eye, soma, crown

protect: Apache Tear, Eilat Stone, Jet, Labradorite, Mohawkite (use as polished stone, make essence by indirect method), Quartz, Richterite, Tantalite, Thunder Egg

remove blockages: Azurite, Bloodstone, Flint, Fulgarite, Green Ridge Quartz, Jasper, Lapis Lazuli, Lemurian Seed, Prehnite with Epidote, Pyrite and Sphalerite, Quartz, Rainbow Mayanite, Rhodozite, Selenite, Serpentine in Obsidian. *Chakra:* dantien

revitalize: Anandalite, Malacholla. *Chakra:* dantien

sacral/navel: Amber, Amphibole, Bastnasite, Blue Jasper, Bumble Bee Jasper, Chinese Red Quartz, Citrine, Clinohumite, Golden Healer Quartz, Keyiapo, Limonite, Orange Calcite, Orange Carnelian, Orange Kyanite, Realgar and Orpiment, Red Jasper, Tangerose, Topaz. Place below navel.

solar plexus: Citrine, Citrine Herkimer, Golden Azeztulite, Golden Beryl, Golden Coracalcite, Golden Danburite, Golden Enhydro, Golden Healer, Green Ridge Quartz, Jasper, Malachite (use as polished stone, make essence by indirect method), Rhodozite, Rhodochrosite, Tangerine Aura Quartz, Tangerine

---

Unless otherwise directed, place crystal in the environment or on a map, apply over an organ or site of symptom, place on an appropriate chakra, wear as jewellery, or bathe with or use as crystal essence.

Dream Lemurian (place above navel), Tiger's Eye, Yellow Tourmaline

soma: Afghanite, Amechlorite, Angelinite, Angel's Wing Calcite, Astraline, Brandenberg Amethyst, Diaspore (Zultanite), Faden Quartz, Holly Agate, Merkabite Calcite, Nuummite, Preseli Bluestone, Stellar Beam Calcite. Place midway on hairline.

Soul Star: Afghanite, Ajoite, Amethyst Elestial, Anandalite™, Angelinite, Angel's Wing Calcite, Astraline, Azeztulite, Brandenberg Amethyst, Diaspore (Zultanite), Golden Himalayan Azeztulite, Green Ridge Quartz, Holly Agate, Merkabite Calcite, Nirvana Quartz, Novaculite, Phenacite in Feldspar, Rosophia, Selenite, Satyaloka Quartz, Satyamani Quartz, Selenite, Stellar Beam Calcite, Titanite (Sphene), White Elestial. Place a foot or so above head.

spleen: Aventurine, Gaspeite, Green Fluorite, Jade, Orange River Quartz, Prasiolite, Rhodonite, Ruby, Zircon. Place below left armpit.

Stellar gateway: Afghanite, Amethyst Elestial, Amphibole, Anandalite™, Angelinite, Angel's Wing Calcite, Astraline, Azeztulite, Brandenberg Amethyst, Diaspore (Zultanite), Fire and Ice, Golden Himalayan Azeztulite, Golden Selenite, Green Ridge Quartz, Holly Agate, Ice Quartz, Merkabite Calcite, Nirvana Quartz, Novaculite, Phenacite, Stellar Beam Calcite,

Unless otherwise directed, place crystal in the environment or on a map, apply over an organ or site of symptom, place on an appropriate chakra, wear as jewellery, or bathe with or use as crystal essence.

Titanite (Sphene), Trigonic Quartz, White Elestial Quartz. Place at arm's length above head.

stimulate or sedate as necessary: Poppy Jasper. *Chakra:* dantien

strengthen: Magnetite (Lodestone), Quartz

third eye: Afghanite, Amechlorite, Ammolite, Apophyllite, Aquamarine, Axinite, Azurite, Black Moonstone, Blue Selenite, Bytownite (Yellow Labradorite), Cacoxenite, Cavansite, Electric-blue Obsidian, Garnet, Glaucophane, Golden Himalayan Azeztulite, Herderite, Herkimer Diamond, Holly Agate, Iolite, Kunzite, Lapis Lazuli, Lavender-purple Opal, Lazulite, Lepidolite, Libyan Gold Tektite, Malachite with Azurite (use as polished stone, make essence by indirect method), Moldavite, Purple Fluorite, Rhomboid Selenite, Royal Sapphire, Serpentine in Obsidian, Sodalite, Spectrolite, Tangerine Aura Quartz. Place above and between eyebrows.

throat: Amber, Amethyst, Aquamarine, Astraline, Azurite, Blue Topaz, Blue Tourmaline, Blue Chalcedony, Blue Lace Agate, Blue Obsidian, Blue Quartz, Chalcanthite, Chrysotile, Glaucophane, Green Ridge Quartz, Indicolite Quartz, Kunzite, Lepidolite, Paraiba Tourmaline, Turquoise. Place over throat.

Cerebellum: Kyanite, Sodalite. *Chakra:* brow, crown

Chemical pollution: Chlorite Quartz, Quantum Quattro,

Unless otherwise directed, place crystal in the environment or on a map, apply over an organ or site of symptom, place on an appropriate chakra, wear as jewellery, or bathe with or use as crystal essence.

Shungite, Smoky Elestial Quartz, Tantalite

Chemotherapy support: Agrellite, Eye of the Storm, Klinoptilolith (wash hands after use, make essence by indirect method), Shungite, Tremolite, Winchite

Chest: Hiddenite, Larimar, Prehnite. *Chakra:* heart

  constriction: Chrysopal (Blue-green Opal), Quantum Quattro

  pains: Amber, Dioptase, Emerald, Malachite (use as polished stone, make essence by indirect method), Rose Quartz, Rhodochrosite, Rhodonite

Cholesterol, high: Aventurine, Magnesite, Yellow Fluorite

Chronic:

  conditions: Apricot Quartz, Bismuth, Diopside

  disease: Apricot Quartz, Bismuth, Cathedral Quartz, Lemurian Jade, Orgonite, Petrified Wood, Quantum Quattro, Que Sera, Shungite, Witches Finger. *Chakra:* dantien

  exhaustion: Apricot Quartz, Bismuth, Bronzite, Cinnabar in Jasper, Eye of the Storm, Poppy Jasper, Prehnite with Epidote, Triplite, Trummer Jasper. *Chakra:* dantien, higher heart

  fatigue syndrome: Adamite, Amethyst, Ametrine, Aquamarine, Apricot Quartz, Aragonite, Barite, Chrysotile in Serpentine, Citrine, Green Tourmaline, Petrified Wood, Pyrite in Quartz, Orange Calcite, Quartz, Rhodochrosite, Ruby, Shungite, Tourmaline,

Triplite, Trummer Jasper, Zincite. *Chakra:* dantien *and see ME* page 221.

illness: Cat's Eye, Danburite, Dendritic Chalcedony, Golden Danburite, Petrified Wood, Poppy Jasper, Que Sera, Shungite, Trummer Jasper. *Chakra:* earth star, solar plexus, higher heart

Circulation: Alabaster, Anglesite, Azurite and Malachite (use as polished stone, make essence by indirect method), Bloodstone, Blue Tiger's Eye, Brazilianite, Brookite, Budd Stone (African Jade), Bustamite, Candle Quartz, Citrine, Clinohumite, Dendritic Agate, Fiskenaesset Ruby, Fulgarite, Garnet in Quartz, Green Diopside, Howlite, Merlinite, Molybdenite, Morion, Ocean Jasper, Ouro Verde, Pyroxmangite, Riebekite with Sugilite and Bustamite, Rosophia, Rhodochrosite, Rose Quartz, Ruby, Stibnite, Thulite, Trigonic Quartz, Yellow Topaz. *Chakra:* dantien, heart

defective: Blue John, Diamond, Garnet, Merlinite, Ruby, Triplite

fortifying: Blue Herkimer with Boulangerite, Pyrope Garnet, Tanzine Aura Quartz

peripheral: Dianite, Ouro Verde, Spangolite

Circulatory:

disorders: Bloodstone, Electric-blue Obsidian, Fulgarite, Hawk's Eye, Hematite, Ruby

system: Amethyst, Bloodstone, Chalcedony, Dendritic Agate, Hematite, Iron Pyrite, Jasper, Magnetite

(Lodestone), Red Jasper

Clearing 'bad vibes': Amazonite, Amber, Amethyst, Aventurine, Black Tourmaline, Chlorite Quartz, Fluorite, Fulgarite, Graphic Smoky Quartz, Iron Pyrite, Kyanite, Lepidolite, Magnetite, Quartz, Smoky Elestial Quartz, Smoky Quartz, Selenite, Shieldite, Shungite, Tantalite, Tektite

Colds: Amethyst, Ametrine, Azurite, Carnelian, Cathedral Quartz, Chalcedony, Emerald, Epidote, Fluorite, Galaxyite, Honey Opal, Hyalite, Kyanite, Labradorite, Larimar, Macedonian Opal, Moss Agate, Ocean Jasper, Orgonite, Quantum Quattro, Que Sera, Rainforest Jasper, Shungite water (drink 2 litres daily), Zoisite. *Chakra:* higher heart

Computer stress: Amazonite, Amber, Aventurine, Chlorite Quartz, Eye of the Storm, Fluorite, Fulgarite, Galena (wash hands after use, make essence by indirect method), Lepidolite, Orgonite, Purple Sugilite, Rose Quartz, Shieldite, Shungite, Smoky Quartz, Sodalite, Sugilite, Tektite. *Chakra:* higher heart

Concentration, improve: Carnelian, Chrysoberyl, Datolite, Diamond, Fluorite, Goethite, Green Tourmaline, Hematite, Herderite, Jade, Lapis Lazuli, Magnetite, Malachite (use as polished stone, make essence by indirect method), Obsidian, Red Jasper, Ruby, Schalenblende. *Chakra:* third eye

Confusion, disperse: Amethyst, Azurite, Bloodstone,

Blue Scapolite, Carnelian, Celestial Quartz, Charoite, Crystal Cap Amethyst, Elestial Quartz, Fluorite, Gabbro, Hematoid Calcite, Howlite, Lapis Lazuli, Lepidocrosite, Limonite, Kakortokite, Magnetite, Opal, Owyhee Blue Opal, Paraiba Tourmaline, Pietersite, Quartz, Rhodochrosite, Sapphire, Selenite, Sodalite. *Chakra:* between third eye and soma

Contraindications and cautions:

bipolar: avoid Rainbow Mayanite, Red Bushman Quartz, Trigonic Quartz

catharsis, may induce: Barite, Epidote, Hypersthene, Smoky Spirit Quartz, Tugtupite (replace with Quantum Quattro or Smoky Quartz)

delicate/sensitive people, may overstimulate: Rainbow Moonstone, Red Bushman Quartz, Scolecite, Tanzanite, Tremolite

depressed: avoid Granite

dizziness, may cause: Preseli Bluestone (change direction)

during full moon: Blue or Rainbow Moonstone – use Black instead

epilepsy: Dumortierite, Goethite, Zircon

giddiness, remove if causes: Banded Agate

headache and nausea, if causes remove: Hanksite (then place Smoky Quartz on earth star)

heart palpitations, if causes remove: Eilat Stone, Malachite (use as polished stone, make essence by indirect method)

hysterical: Red Bushman Quartz

illusion, may induce: Blue or Rainbow Moonstone

insomnia: Do not wear Herkimer Diamond earrings or place on third eye, avoid Rose Quartz by the bed.

negative energy heightened if worn constantly: Epidote, Hypersthene

pacemakers: Zircon may cause dizziness

Preseli Bluestone:. Do not place in bedroom overnight.

psychiatric conditions, paranoia or schizophrenia: Do not use crystals unless under the supervision of a qualified crystal healer.

radioactive: very dark Smoky Quartz, Uranophane

sensitive people: Tanzanite may overstimulate psychic abilities as may Rainbow or Blue Moonstone (use black or pink Moonstone instead)

Tanzanite/Blue Moonstone/Rainbow Moonstone may create uncontrolled psychic experiences or mental overload, or unwanted telepathy

toehold in incarnation: avoid Gabbro with Moonstone, Llanite (Llanoite), Polychrome Jasper.
Chakra: earth star and soma

toxic, may contain traces of toxic minerals although these are bound up within the structure (use polished stone where possible, make crystal essence by indirect method, wash hands after handling):

Unless otherwise directed, place crystal in the environment or on a map, apply over an organ or site of symptom, place on an appropriate chakra, wear as jewellery, or bathe with or use as crystal essence.

Actinolite, Adamite, Andaluscite, Ajoite, Alexandrite, Almandine Garnet, Amazonite, Aquamarine, Aragonite, Arsenopyrite, Atacamite, Aurichalcite, Axinite, Azurite, Beryl, Beryllium, Biotite (ferrous), Bixbite, Black Tourmaline, Boji Stones, Bornite, Brazilianite, Brochantite, Bumble Bee Jasper, Cassiterite, Cavansite, Celestite, Cerussite, Cervanite, Chalcanthite, Chalcopyrite (Peacock Ore), Chrysoberyl, Chrysocolla, Chrysotile, Cinnabar, Conichalcite, Copper, Covellite, Crocoite, Cryolite, Cuprite, Diopside, Dioptase, Dumortierite, Emerald, Epidote, Garnet, Gem Silica, Galena, Garnierite (Falcondoite), Germanium, Goshenite, Heliodor, Hessonite Garnet, Hiddenite, Jadeite, Jamesonite, Iolite, Kinoite, Klinoptilolith, Kunzite, Kyanite, Labradorite, Lapis Lazuli, Lazurite, Lepidolite, Magnetite, Malachite, Malacholla, Marcasite, Messina Quartz, Mohawkite, Moldavite, Moonstone, Moqui Balls, Morganite, Orpiment, Pargasite, Piemontite, Pietersite, Plancheite, Prehnite, Psilomelane, Pyrite, Pyromorphite, Quantum Quattro, Que Sera, Realgar, Realgar and Orpiment, Renierite, Rhodolite Garnet, Ruby, Sapphire, Serpentine, Smithsonite, Sodalite, Spessartine Garnet, Sphalerite, Spinel, Spodumene, Staurolite, Stibnite, Stilbite, Suglite, Sulphur, Sunstone, Tanzanite, Tiffany Stone, Tiger's Eye, Topaz, Torbernite, Tourmaline, Tremolite, Turquoise,

Unless otherwise directed, place crystal in the environment or on a map, apply over an organ or site of symptom, place on an appropriate chakra, wear as jewellery, or bathe with or use as crystal essence.

Uranophane, Uvarovite Garnet, Valentinite, Vanadinite, Variscite, Vesuvianite, Vivianite, Wavellite, Wulfenite, Zircon, Zoisite

Convalescence: Bixbite, Brandenberg Amethyst, Chohua Jasper, Empowerite, Epidote, Macedonian Opal, Nzuri Moyo, Quantum Quattro, Que Sera, Stichtite, Victorite. Wear constantly.

Core:

energy: Erythrite, Lemurian Jade, Menalite, Poppy Jasper, Silver Leaf Jasper, Smoky Rose Quartz, Trummer Jasper. *Chakra:* dantien

strength/stability: Crinoidal Limestone, Eye of the Storm, Flint, Golden Healer Quartz, Hematite, Mohawkite (use as polished stone, make essence by indirect method), Polychrome Jasper

Cramp: Amethyst, Bloodstone, Malachite (use as polished stone, make essence by indirect method), Magnesite, Magnetite (Lodestone), Obsidian, Serpentine, Smoky Quartz, Turquoise, Zircon

intestinal: Green Fluorite, Magnesite

legs: Hematite, Lepidolite

muscles: Magnetite (Lodestone)

release: Azurite with Malachite (use as polished stone, make essence by indirect method), Cathedral Quartz, Mohawkite (use as polished stone, make essence by indirect method)

stomach: Magnesite

Unless otherwise directed, place crystal in the environment or on a map, apply over an organ or site of symptom, place on an appropriate chakra, wear as jewellery, or bathe with or use as crystal essence.

Creativity, improve: Amethyst Herkimer, Bixbite, Blue Quartz, Bushman Quartz, Covellite, Eilat Stone, Girasol, Greenlandite, Icicle Calcite, Quantum Quattro, Rain Forest Jasper, Septarian, Seriphos Quartz, Tangerine Sun Aura Quartz, Triplite. *Chakra:* sacral, dantien

'Cure all': Clear Calcite, Eye of the Storm, Golden Healer Quartz, Poppy Jasper, Quantum Quattro, Quartz, Que Sera, Shungite. *Chakra:* dantien, higher heart, third eye. Or wear continuously.

- D -

Dark moods, ameliorate: Kunzite, Rutilated Quartz. *Chakra:* solar plexus, brow

Decision making:

    overcome inability in: Azurite, Green Tourmaline, Rutilated Quartz

    overcome indecision: Azurite, Blue Fluorite, Bronzite, Bytownite, Charoite, Covellite, Crazy Lace Agate, Cryolite, Diamond, Emerald, Eye of the Storm, Golden Healer Quartz, Green Tourmaline, Hawk's Eye, Jade, Lepidolite, Poppy Jasper, Rutilated Quartz, Tiger's Eye, Yellow Scapolite. *Chakra:* dantien

Debility: Black Tourmaline, Fire Agate. *Chakra:* base

Degenerative disease: Ammolite, Brown Jasper, Budd Stone (African Jade), Citrine, Holly Agate, Moonstone, Nuummite, Pearl, Ruby, Scolecite with Natrolite, Stichtite. *Chakra:* dantien, higher heart

Dementia: Anthrophyllite, Atlantasite, Holly Agate, Stichtite, Stichtite and Serpentine. *Chakra:* third eye, alta major

Depression: Ajo Blue Calcite, Amber, Amethyst, Ametrine, Apatite, Apophyllite, Botswana Agate, Carnelian, Chrysoprase, Citrine, Clinohumite, Dianite, Eisenkiesel, Eudialyte, Flint, Garnet, Golden Healer, Green Ridge Quartz, Hematite, Idocrase, Jade, Jet, Kunzite, Lapis Lazuli, Lepidolite, Lithium Quartz,

Unless otherwise directed, place crystal in the environment or on a map, apply over an organ or site of symptom, place on an appropriate chakra, wear as jewellery, or bathe with or use as crystal essence.

Macedonian Opal, Maw Sit Sit, Montebrasite, Moss Agate, Orange Kyanite, Pink Sunstone, Porphyrite (Chinese Letter Stone), Purple Tourmaline, Rainbow Goethite, Rutilated Quartz, Siberian Quartz, Sillimanite, Smoky Quartz, Spessartine Garnet, Spinel, Spider Web Obsidian, Staurolite, Sunstone, Tiger's Eye, Tugtupite, Turquoise. *Chakra:* solar plexus. Wear continuously.

Dermatitis: Snakeskin Agate, Wavellite

Despair: Candle Quartz, Carnelian, Eye of the Storm, Golden Healer Quartz, Iron Pyrite, Novaculite, Pyrite in Quartz, Rhodonite, Serpentine, Sugilite, Vera Cruz Amethyst. *Chakra:* heart. Wear continuously.

Despondency: Candle Quartz, Harlequin Quartz, Purpurite. *Chakra:* heart

Detoxification: Amber, Amechlorite, Amethyst, Anhydrite, Apache Tear, Aventurine, Azurite, Banded Agate, Barite, Bastnasite, Bloodstone, Chalk, Chlorite, Chlorite Quartz, Chrysoprase, Conichalcite, Coprolite, Covellite, Cuprite with Chrysocolla, Dendritic Agate, Diaspore, Emerald, Eye of the Storm, Fire Obsidian, Galena (wash hands after use, make essence by indirect method), Golden Danburite, Golden Healer Quartz, Graphic Smoky Quartz, Green Garnet, Greensand, Halite, Hanksite, Herkimer Diamond, Hypersthene, Iolite, Jade, Jamesonite, Jet, Kambaba Jasper, Larvikite, Malachite (use as polished stone, make essence by indirect method), Merlinite, Mica, Obsidian, Ocean

Jasper, Orgonite, Phlogopite, Poppy Jasper, Pumice, Quantum Quattro, Que Sera, Rainbow Covellite, Richterite, Ruby, Seraphinite, Shungite, Smoky Elestial Quartz, Smoky Quartz, Smoky Quartz with Aegerine, Stilbite, Sulphur, Sulphur in Quartz, Thunder Egg, Tiger's Eye, Topaz, Tree Agate, Turquoise, Zoisite. *Chakra:* solar plexus, earth star, base. Or place in environment.

Diabetes/blood sugar imbalances: Angel's Wing Calcite, Astraline, Atlantasite, Bastnasite, Bowenite (New Jade), Chinese Chromium Quartz, Chrome Diopside, Chrysolite in Serpentine, Citrine, Datolite, Diamond (worn at waist, on left side, as close to the pancreas as possible), Emerald, Huebnerite, Jade, Malacholla, Malachite (use as polished stone, make essence by indirect method), Maw Sit Sit, Mtrolite, Owyhee Blue Opal, Pink Opal, Quantum Quattro, Que Sera, Red Jasper, Red Serpentine, Schalenblende, Serpentine, Serpentine in Obsidian, Shungite, Stichtite, Stichtite with Serpentine, Tugtupite, and see Blood sugar page 162 and Pancreas page 230. *Chakra*: dantien, spleen

Diarrhoea: Green Tourmaline, Lapis Lazuli, Malachite (use as polished stone, make essence by indirect method), Pearl, Quartz, Serpentine

Digestion: Amblygonite, Chrysocolla, Citrine, Coprolite, Covellite, Golden Selenite, Iron Pyrite, Labradorite, Leopardskin Jasper, Limonite, Morion, Mystic Topaz, Obsidian, Ocean Jasper, Peridot Rhodonite, Sapphire,

Smithsonite, Snowflake Obsidian, Steatite, Tiger's Eye, Topaz, Yellow Apatite. *Chakra:* solar plexus, dantien

    calm: Chrysocolla, Chrysoprase, Green Jasper, Iron Pyrite

    faulty: Red Tourmaline, Yellow Jasper

    stimulate: Moss Agate, Red Jade

    strengthen: Iron Pyrite

Digestive:

    organs, problems: Anthrophyllite, Klinoptilolith (wash hands after use, make essence by indirect method), Shungite. Place over site.

    organs, strengthen: Bustamite, Empowerite, Fire Agate, Jasper, Kambaba Jasper, Montebrasite, Pyrite in Quartz, Serpentine in Obsidian, Shungite, Snakeskin Pyrite, Topaz. *Chakra:* dantien, solar plexus

    tract: Amethyst, Anthrophyllite, Cat's Eye Quartz, Chrysocolla, Crackled Fire Agate, Pink Tourmaline, Serpentine in Obsidian

Disconnection from Earth: Flint, Granite, Hematite, Lemurian Jade, Libyan Gold Tektite, Preseli Bluestone, Quartz, Smoky Elestial Quartz, Strontianite, Tektite and see Grounding page 201. *Chakra:* dantien, soma

Dis-ease due to stress: Amechlorite, Basalt, Bird's Eye Jasper, Black Moonstone, Eye of the Storm, Galaxyite, Lemurian Gold Opal, Macedonian Opal, Marble, Orgonite, Richterite, Riebekite with Sugilite and Bustamite, Shungite, Tektite, Tugtupite and see Stress

Dizziness: Aragonite, Candle Quartz, Cathedral Quartz, Dioptase, Eye of the Storm, Flint, Golden Healer Quartz, Hematite, Lapis Lazuli, Mohawkite (use as polished stone, make essence by indirect method), Poppy Jasper, Quartz, Richterite, White Sapphire. *Chakra:* dantien, crown

191

Unless otherwise directed, place crystal in the environment or on a map, apply over an organ or site of symptom, place on an appropriate chakra, wear as jewellery, or bathe with or use as crystal essence.

- E -

Earth, attune to: Chrysocolla, Granite, Hematite, Hiddenite, Preseli Bluestone

Earth healing: Ammolite, Aragonite, Black Diopside, Black Tourmaline, Blue Sapphire, Brown Aragonite, Bustamite, Cacoxenite, Celestial Quartz, Champagne Aura Quartz, Chlorite Quartz, Desert Rose, Dragon Stone, Eye of the Storm, Feldspar, Flint, Fulgarite, Golden or Tangerine Lemurian, Green Ridge Quartz, Kambaba Jasper, Granite, Greenlandite, Labradorite, Lemurian Jade, Marble, Mohawkite (use as polished stone, make essence by indirect method), Monazite, Prehnite, Preseli Bluestone, Quartz, Rhodozite, Scolecite, Selenite, Seriphos Quartz, Smoky Brandenberg, Smoky Elestial, Smoky Quartz, Specular Hematite, Stromatolite, Super 7, Tantalite, Thunder Egg, Torbernite, Witches Finger, Z-stone. *Chakra:* earth star, place in environment

Eczema: Amethyst, Green Aventurine, Sapphire. Bathe with alcohol-free crystal essence.

Electrical systems of body, rebalance: Amber, Amblygonite, Cavansite, Galena (wash hands after use, make essence by indirect method), Golden Healer Quartz, Montebrasite, Orgonite, Pollucite, Shiva Lingam, Shungite

Electrolytes, nerve and muscle function: Coral, Malachite (use as polished stone, make essence by

---

Unless otherwise directed, place crystal in the environment or on a map, apply over an organ or site of symptom, place on an appropriate chakra, wear as jewellery, or bathe with or use as crystal essence.

indirect method), Native Copper, Quartz

Electromagnetic:

> **antidote:** Ajoite in Shattuckite, Amazonite, Amber, Aventurine, Auralite 23, Black Moonstone, Black Tourmaline, Black Tourmaline in Quartz, Blizzard Stone, Bloodstone, Chlorite Quartz, Diamond, Flint, Fluorite, Fluorapatite, Fulgarite, Gabbro, Galena (wash hands after use, make essence by indirect method), Graphic Smoky Quartz, Herkimer Diamond, Jasper, Klinoptilolith (wash hands after use, make essence by indirect method), Lepidolite, Malachite (use as polished stone, make essence by indirect method), Native Copper, Natrolite, Obsidian, Orgonite, Phlogopite, Pollucite, Pyrite in Quartz, Quartz, Quantum Quattro, Que Sera, Red Amethyst, Rose Quartz, Scolecite, Shieldite, Shungite, Smoky Quartz, Sodalite, Stilbite, Thomsonite, Thunder Egg, Yellow Kunzite

> **field, regulate personal:** Ajoite in Shattuckite, Amazonite, Amber, Auralite 23, Black Moonstone, Champagne Aura Quartz, Eye of the Storm, Fluorapatite, Fluorite, Fulgarite, Gabbro, Galena (wash hands after use, make essence by indirect method), Golden Healer Quartz, Montebrasite, Poppy Jasper, Preseli Bluestone, Quantum Quattro, Que Sera, Rose Quartz, Shungite. *Chakra:* earth star, base. Or place in environment.

Unless otherwise directed, place crystal in the environment or on a map, apply over an organ or site of symptom, place on an appropriate chakra, wear as jewellery, or bathe with or use as crystal essence.

pollution, protect against: Ajoite in Shattuckite, Amazonite, Amber, Andara Glass, Black Moonstone, Black Tourmaline, Blizzard Stone, Champagne Aura Quartz, Chlorite Quartz, Diamond, Flint, Fluorite, Gabbro, Galena (wash hands after use, make essence by indirect method), Graphic Smoky Quartz, Hackmanite, Herkimer Diamond, Klinoptilolith (wash hands after use, make essence by indirect method), Kunzite, Lepidolite, Malachite (use as polished stone, make essence by indirect method), Marble, Morion, Native Copper, Orgonite, Phlogopite, Poppy Jasper, Quartz, Que Sera, Red Amethyst, Rose Quartz, Shieldite, Shungite, Smoky Elestial Quartz, Smoky Herkimer Diamond, Smoky Quartz, Sodalite, Tantalite, Thunder Egg. *Chakra:* earth star, base. Or place in environment or around house.

Emphysema: Amber, Amethyst, Aqua Aura, Dioptase, Emerald, Kambaba Jasper, Malachite (use as polished stone, make essence by indirect method), Morganite, Rhodonite, Rose Quartz, Stromatolite, Tiger's Eye

Endocrine system: Amber, Amethyst, Adamite, Alexandrite, Amechlorite, Aquamarine, Azeztulite with Morganite, Black Moonstone, Bloodstone, Blue Quartz, Bustamite, Champagne Aura Quartz, Chrysoberyl, Citrine, Fire Agate, Fire and Ice Quartz, Golden Healer, Golden Topaz, Green Calcite, Green Obsidian, Howlite, Magnetite, Menalite, Pargasite, Pentagonite, Peridot,

Picrolite, Pietersite, Pink Heulandite, Pink Tourmaline, Poppy Jasper, Quantum Quattro, Que Sera, Rhodochrosite, Richterite, Ruby Aura Quartz, Seriphos Quartz, Smoky Amethyst, Sodalite, Strummer Jasper, Topaz, Tourmaline, Yellow Jasper. *Chakra:* dantien, higher heart

Endurance, boost: Chalcedony, Jade, Honey Phantom Calcite, Poppy Jasper, Septarian, Triplite. *Chakra:* base, sacral, dantien

Energetic well-being: Cinnabar Jasper, Fire Agate, Golden Healer Quartz, Jamesonite, Poppy Jasper, Quantum Quattro, Que Sera, Strummer Jasper, Tantalite

Energy: Agate, Amber, Apophyllite, Aragonite, Bloodstone, Blue Goldstone, Calcite, Carnelian, Coral, Danburite, Fire Agate, Green Jasper, Hematite, Jasper, Peridot, Prehnite, Quartz, Quantum Quattro, Que Sera, Rhodochrosite, Ruby, Rutilated Quartz, Strawberry Lemurian, Triplite. *Chakra:* base, sacral, dantien. Or place in environment.

> **amplify:** Poppy Jasper, Preseli Bluestone, Ruby Lavender Quartz, Sedona Stone, Triplite. *Chakra:* base, dantien

> **blockages:** Charoite, Danburite, Flint, Fulgarite, Labradorite, Lemurian Quartz

> **depletion, reverse:** Eudialyte, Fire Opal, Macedonian Opal, Pink Sunstone, Poppy Jasper, Preseli Bluestone, Que Sera, Red Jasper, Ruby Lavender Quartz,

Rutilated Quartz, Scheelite, Sedona Stone, Strawberry Lemurian. *Chakra:* dantien

energetic cleanse: Amber, Anandalite, Merlinite

field, strengthen: Garnet, Kunzite, Mohawkite (use as polished stone, make essence by indirect method), Poppy Jasper, Preseli Bluestone, Quartz, Ruby Lavender Quartz. *Chakra:* dantien, solar plexus

imbalances: Lepidocrosite

leakage from aura: Amber, Flint, Healer's Gold, Labradorite, Molybdenite in Quartz, Nuummite, Pyrite in Quartz, Strawberry Lemurian, Rainbow Mayanite, Tantalite. *Chakra:* dantien, higher heart

stagnant: Black Tourmaline, Calcite, Clear Topaz, Graphic Smoky Quartz, Smoky Elestial Quartz, Smoky Quartz

system: Garnet in Quartz. *Chakra:* dantien

unbalanced field: Amber, Garnet in Quartz, Goldsheen Obsidian, Preseli Bluestone, Ruby in Zoisite

Environment, improve: Aragonite, Amazonite, Black Tourmaline, Chlorite Quartz, Eye of the Storm, Golden Healer Quartz, Malachite (use as polished stone, make essence by indirect method), Orgonite, Quartz, Poppy Jasper, Rose Quartz, Selenite, Smoky Quartz, White or Rose Elestial Quartz and see Earth healing page 192

Environmental:

diseases: Chlorite Quartz, Drusy Quartz on

Sphalerite, Eye of the Storm, Feldspar, Golden Healer Quartz, Marble, Orgonite, Petrified Wood, Poppy Jasper, Preseli Bluestone, Quartz, Shieldite, Shungite, Smoky Elestial Quartz, and see Geopathic stress page 201. *Chakra:* earth star. Or place in environment.

harmony: Khutnohorite, Rose Quartz, Sardonyx, Selenite

pollution: Alunite, Amber, Anhydrite, Black Tourmaline, Champagne Aura Quartz, Chlorite Quartz, Eye of the Storm, Flint, Golden Healer Quartz, Graphic Smoky Quartz, Halite, Hanksite, Labradorite, Moss Agate, Orgonite, Phlogopite, Poppy Jasper, Que Sera, Selenite, Shieldite, Shungite, Smoky Elestial Quartz, Smoky Quartz, Sulphur, Sulphur in Quartz, Tantalite, Thunder Egg, Trummer Jasper, Zincite. *Chakra:* earth star. Place stones in earth or around house.

Eruptions on skin: Faden Quartz, Honey Calcite, Klinoptilolith (wash hands after use, make essence by indirect method), Riebekite with Sugilite and Bustamite, Snakeskin Agate, Sulphur in Quartz, Wind Fossil Agate

Etheric:

blueprint: Andescine Labradorite, Angelinite, Astraline, Brandenberg Amethyst, Chlorite Quartz, Chrysotile, Elestial Quartz, Ethiopian Opal, Eye of the Storm, Flint, Girasol, Keyiapo, Khutnohorite, Lemurian Aquitane Calcite, Rhodozite, Ruby

Lavender Quartz, Sanda Rosa Azeztulite, Scheelite, Stellar Beam Calcite, Tangerine Dream Lemurian, Tantalite. *Chakra:* past life

body: Ethiopian Opal, Golden Selenite and see Aura page 156

Etheric bodies/biomagnetic field, realign/strengthen: Angelinite, Astraline, Ethiopian Opal, Gold in Quartz, Golden Healer Quartz, Poldarvaarite, Pollucite, Quantum Quattro, Que Sera

Exhaustion: Bismuth, Carnelian, Chlorite Quartz, Cinnabar Jasper, Cuprite with Chrysocolla, Epidote, Eye of the Storm, Fire Opal, Garnet, Golden Healer Quartz, Hematite, Lepidolite, Pietersite, Poppy Jasper, Quantum Quattro, Red Jasper, Ruby, Rutilated Quartz, Scheelite, Sulphur, Tiger Iron, Triplite, Turquoise. *Chakra:* base

- F -

Family:

> **stress:** Candle Quartz, Chinese Red Quartz, Datolite, Eye of the Storm, Faden Quartz, Fairy Quartz, Glendonite, Mohave Turquoise, Riebekite with Sugilite and Bustamite, Selenite, Shaman Quartz, Shungite, Spirit Quartz. *Chakra:* solar plexus

Fatigue: Amethyst, Ametrine, Bloodstone, Blue Opal, Carnelian, Dendritic Agate, Dioptase, Galena (wash hands after use, make essence by indirect method), Hematite, Iron Pyrite, Rose Quartz, Staurolite, Sunstone, Triplite

Female reproductive system: Amber, Carnelian, Chrysoprase, Malachite (use as polished stone, make essence by indirect method), Menalite, Moonstone, Topaz, Unakite, Wulfenite. *Chakra:* sacral, base

Fertility: Basalt, Cinnabar Jasper, Golden Healer Quartz, Menalite, Orange Kyanite

> **increase:** Atacamite, Calcite Fairy Stone, Carnelian, Dragon Stone, Jade, Menalite, Moonstone, Orange Kyanite, Orange Sapphire, Rose Quartz, Ruby in Zoisite, Tree Agate, Triplite, Tugtupite. *Chakra:* sacral, dantien

Fluid: Eye of the Storm, Moonstone, Nunderite, Oligocrase, Trigonic Quartz. *Chakra:* dantien, solar plexus

---

Unless otherwise directed, place crystal in the environment or on a map, apply over an organ or site of symptom, place on an appropriate chakra, wear as jewellery, or bathe with or use as crystal essence.

deficiency: Moonstone, Trigonic Quartz

excess: Brochantite, Diamond, Halite, Jade, Rose Quartz, Scheelite, Smoky Amethyst

imbalances: Azeztulite with Morganite, Bastnasite, Eye of the Storm, Hackmanite, Jade, Mookaite Jasper, Moonstone, Nunderite, Oligocrase, Rainforest Jasper, Scheelite, Trigonic Quartz

retention: Amber, Andean Opal, Aqua Aura, Aquamarine, Bastnasite, Bustamite, Chalcanthite, Chalcedony, Chrysoprase, Cuprite with Chrysocolla, Diaspore (Zultanite), Eye of the Storm, Greensand, Hackmanite, Halite, Hanksite, Jade, Mookaite Jasper, Moonstone, Nunderite, Opalised Fossilised Wood, Pearl, Quartz, Scheelite, Smoky Amethyst, Sonora Sunrise, Trigonic Quartz. *Chakra:* solar plexus

Forgetfulness: Chlorite Quartz, Emerald, Eye of the Storm, Golden Healer Quartz, Moss Agate, Poppy Jasper, Rhodonite, Sodalite, Tourmaline, Unakite. *Chakra:* brow

Free radicals:

damage from: Brochantite, Diaspore (Zultanite), Klinoptilolith (wash hands after use, make essence by indirect method), Selenite, Shungite. *Chakra:* higher heart

remove: Diaspore, Klinoptilolith (wash hands after use, make essence by indirect method), Piemontite, Shungite

---

Unless otherwise directed, place crystal in the environment or on a map, apply over an organ or site of symptom, place on an appropriate chakra, wear as jewellery, or bathe with or use as crystal essence.

- G -

Gastric:
  ulcer: Shungite. *Chakra:* solar plexus
  upset: Shungite. *Chakra:* solar plexus
Gastric disturbance causing insomnia: Hackmanite, Khutnohorite, Pyrite in Quartz, Shungite. *Chakra:* solar plexus
Gastritis: Shungite
Geopathic stress: Amazonite, Amethyst, Black Tourmaline, Brown Jasper, Champagne Aura Quartz, Chlorite Quartz, Eye of the Storm, Flint, Gabbro, Granite, Graphic Smoky Quartz, Ironstone, Kunzite, Labradorite, Marble, Orgonite, Preseli Bluestone, Pyrite and Sphalerite, Quartz, Riebekite with Sugilite and Bustamite, Selenite, Shieldite, Shungite, Smoky Amethyst, Smoky Elestial, Smoky Quartz, Sodalite, Strummer Jasper, Tantalite, Tektite, Thunder Egg. *Chakra:* earth star. Or place around corners of house.
Giddiness: Boji Stones, Emerald, Hematite, Pearl, Quartz, Sodalite. *Chakra:* dantien
Grounding: Ajo Quartz, Amphibole, Aztee, Blue Aragonite, Boji Stones, Bronzite, Bustamite, Calcite Fairy Stone, Champagne Aura Quartz, Chlorite Quartz, Cloudy Quartz, Dalmatian Stone, Empowerite, Flint, Gabbro, Healer's Gold, Hematite, Hematoid Calcite, Herkimer Diamond, Honey Phantom Quartz, Jasper,

Kambaba Jasper, Keyiapo, Lazulite, Lemurian Jade, Lemurian Seed, Leopardskin Serpentine, Libyan Gold Tektite, Limonite, Madagascar Cloudy Quartz, Mahogany Obsidian, Marcasite, Merlinite, Mohawkite (use as polished stone, make essence by indirect method), Novaculite, Nunderite, Peanut Wood, Pearl Spa Dolomite, Petrified Wood, Poppy Jasper, Preseli Bluestone, Purpurite, Pyrite in Magnesite, Quantum Quattro, Rutile with Hematite, Schalenblende, Serpentine in Obsidian, Smoky Elestial Quartz, Smoky Quartz, Smoky Herkimer, Sodalite, Steatite, Stromatolite. *Chakra:* base, earth star, dantien

- H -

Headache: Amber, Amblygonite, Blue Sapphire, Bustamite, Cathedral Quartz, Champagne Aura Quartz, Dioptase, Dumortierite, Galena (wash hands after use, make essence by indirect method), Greenlandite, Hematite, Jet, Lapis Lazuli, Magnesite, Pyrite in Magnesite, Quantum Quattro, Rhodozite, Rose Quartz, Smoky Quartz, Sugilite, Turquoise. *Chakra:* third eye

arising from:

blocked alta major chakra: Blue Moonstone, Garnet in Pyroxene, Herderite, Orange Kyanite, Riebekite with Sugilite and Bustamite, and see Alta Major chakra page 172

neck tension: Cathedral Quartz, Magnetite (Lodestone), Quantum Quattro. On base of skull.

negative environmental factors/electromagnetic stress: Galena (wash hands after use, make essence by indirect method), Smoky Quartz, Tektite. See Electromagnetic stress page 193 and Geopathic stress page 201.

Heart: Adamite, Andean Blue Opal, Brandenberg Amethyst, Blue or Green Aventurine, Bustamite, Cacoxenite, Candle Quartz, Fiskenaesset Ruby, Garnet, Garnet in Quartz, Golden Danburite, Green Diopside, Green Heulandite, Green Obsidian, Holly Agate, Khutnohorite, Merlinite, Peridot, Picrolite, Pink or

Watermelon Tourmaline, Prasiolite, Quantum Quattro, Rhodochrosite, Rhodonite, Rose Quartz, Rose Elestial Quartz, Rosophia, Sapphire, Tugtupite and see Heart chakra page 175. *Chakra:* heart

> **attacks:** Aventurine, Dioptase, Gaspeite, Tantalite, Tugtupite
>
> **beat, irregular:** Dumortierite, Jade, Rhodochrosite
>
> **burn:** Carnelian, Dioptase, Emerald, Montebrasite, Peridot, Pyrope Garnet, Pyrophyllite, Quartz
>
> **chakra:** see Chakras page 171
>
> **disease:** Carnelian, Eudialyte, Hemimorphite, Morganite, Red Jasper, Rhodochrosite, Rhodonite, Ruby, Smoky Amethyst, Tourmalinated Quartz, Tugtupite
>
> **failure:** Scheelite
>
> **healer:** Azeztulite with Morganite, Khutnohorite, Pyroxmangite, Rhodozaz, Roselite, Rosophia
>
> **inflammation:** Blue Euclase, Hematite, Pink Lemurian Seed, Rhodozite, Sulphur in Quartz, Zoisite
>
> **invigorate:** Chohua Jasper, Green Garnet, Lemurian Jade
>
> **muscle:** Kunzite, Septarian
>
> **rhythm, disturbed:** Brandenberg Amethyst, Honey Calcite, Serpentine
>
> **strengthen:** Calcite, Chohua Jasper, Danburite, Erythrite, Honey Calcite, Lemurian Jade, Pink Lemurian Seed, Rose Quartz, Strawberry Quartz,

Tugtupite

trauma, heal: Azeztulite with Morganite, Blue Euclase, Cobalto Calcite, Gaia Stone, Larimar, Mangano Vesuvianite, Oceanite, Peanut Wood, Quantum Quattro, Rose Elestial Quartz, Roselite, Ruby Lavender Quartz, Tantalite, Victorite

unblock: Dioptase, Gaspeite, Pink Lemurian Seed, Prasiolite, Rose Quartz, Smoky Rose Quartz

High frequency communication aerials, microwaves, infrared and radar: Amazonite, Amethyst, Black Moonstone, Black Tourmaline, Chlorite Quartz, Fluorite, Gabbro, Germanium, Granite, Graphic Smoky Quartz, Hematite, Herkimer Diamond, Klinoptilolith (wash hands after use, make essence by indirect method), Malachite (use as polished stone, make essence by indirect method), Orgonite, Reinerite, Shieldite, Shungite, Smoky Elestial Quartz, Smoky Quartz, Sodalite, Sphalerite, Tourmaline, Tourmalinated Quartz, Yellow Kunzite, Zeolite. Place around site or between you and the site.

Homeostasis: Enstatite and Diopside, Klinoptilolith (wash hands after use, make essence by indirect method), Piemontite, Quantum Quattro, Reinerite. *Chakra:* dantien

maintain: Klinoptilolith (wash hands after use, make essence by indirect method), Piemontite, Shungite

Hormones: see also Endocrine system page 194

Unless otherwise directed, place crystal in the environment or on a map, apply over an organ or site of symptom, place on an appropriate chakra, wear as jewellery, or bathe with or use as crystal essence.

boosting: Amechlorite, Amethyst, Cassiterite, Lepidolite, Menalite, Paraiba Tourmaline, Pietersite, Smoky Amethyst. *Chakra:* third eye, higher heart

imbalances: Amechlorite, Astrophyllite, Black Moonstone, Champagne Aura Quartz, Chinese Chromium Quartz, Chrysoprase, Citrine, Diopside, Hemimorphite, Labradorite, Menalite, Moonstone, Paraiba Tourmaline, Sonora Sunrise, Tanzine Aura Quartz, Tugtupite. *Chakra:* third eye, higher heart

regulate: Champagne Aura Quartz, Chinese Chromium Quartz, Menalite, Smoky Amethyst, Tugtupite, Watermelon Tourmaline. *Chakra:* brow, higher heart

Hyperactivity: Black Moonstone, Cerussite, Cumberlandite, Dianite, Fiskenaesset Ruby, Garnet, Green Tourmaline, Lepidocrosite, Montebrasite, Moonstone, Pearl Spa Dolomite, Yellow Scapolite. *Chakra:* earth star, base, dantien

Hypersensitivity: Dumortierite, Proustite and see Oversensitive page 229

Hypertension: Apatite

Hyperthyroidism: Atacamite, Cacoxenite, Champagne Aura Quartz, Cryolite, Richterite, Tanzine Aura Quartz. *Chakra:* throat Quartz (or wear continuously)

Hypoglycaemia: Atlantasite, Bowenite (New Jade), Datolite, Maw Sit Sit, Pink Opal, Schalenblende, Stichtite and Serpentine, Tugtupite and see Pancreas page 230.

Unless otherwise directed, place crystal in the environment or on a map, apply over an organ or site of symptom, place on an appropriate chakra, wear as jewellery, or bathe with or use as crystal essence.

Chakra: dantien, spleen

Hypothalamus: Blue Moonstone, Preseli Bluestone, Richterite, Tanzine Aura Quartz

Immune system: Agate, Amechlorite, Anandalite™, Ametrine, Black or Green Tourmaline, Blue Agate, Brown Jasper, Bloodstone, Carnelian, Chevron Amethyst, Chohua Jasper, Chiastolite, Diaspore (Zultanite), Emerald, Fuchsite, Fuchsite with Ruby, Green Calcite, Klinoptilolith (wash hands after use, make essence by indirect method), Kunzite, Lapis Lazuli, Lemurian Jade, Lepidolite, Macedonian Green Opal, Malachite (use as polished stone, make essence by indirect method), Moss Agate, Mookaite Jasper, Nzuri Moyo, Ocean Jasper, Paraiba Tourmaline, Pentagonite, Petrified Wood, Preseli Bluestone, Quantum Quattro, Quartz, Que Sera, Reinerite, Richterite, Rosophia, Ruby in Zoisite, Seriphos Quartz, Schalenblende, Shungite, Smithsonite, Smoky Quartz with Aegerine, Super 7, Tangerose, Titanite (Sphene), Thunder Egg, Tourmaline, Turquoise, Winchite, Zoisite. *Chakra:* dantien, higher heart. Place around corners of bed.

Impotence: Basalt, Bastnasite, Carnelian, Cinnabar Jasper, Garnet, Morganite, Orange Kyanite, Poppy Jasper, Rhodonite, Sodalite, Shiva Lingam, Triplite, Variscite. *Chakra:* base, sacral

Indigestion: Candle Quartz, Chalk, Citrine, Jasper, Peridot, Tourmaline. *Chakra:* solar plexus

Infection: Amethyst, Blue Lace Agate, Galena (wash hands after use, make essence by indirect method), Green

---

Unless otherwise directed, place crystal in the environment or on a map, apply over an organ or site of symptom, place on an appropriate chakra, wear as jewellery, or bathe with or use as crystal essence.

Calcite, Kunzite, Malachite (use as polished stone, make essence by indirect method), Moss Agate, Opal, Quantum Quattro, Que Sera, Shungite, Smoky Quartz, Sulphur (spray room with crystal essence made by indirect method), Sulphur in Quartz. *Chakra:* higher heart or place in environment

    acute: Bloodstone, Chrysocolla, Quantum Quattro, Rhodochrosite, Shungite, Sulphur (use as polished crystallized stone, make essence by indirect method)

    increase resistance to: Amethyst, Quantum Quattro, Que Sera, Shungite. Wear continuously.

Infertility: Banded Agate, Bastnasite, Bixbite, Blue Euclase, Brookite, 'Citrine' Herkimer, Eye of the Storm, Fiskenaesset Ruby, Garnet, Granite, Menalite, Moonstone, Poppy Jasper, Shiva Lingam, Spirit Quartz, Thulite, Triplite, Tugtupite, Zincite. *Chakra:* base and sacral and see Fertility page 199

Inflammation/inflamed joints: Bloodstone, Blue Chalcedony, Blue Euclase, Blue Lace Agate, Brochantite, Cathedral Quartz, Chalcopyrite, Chrysocolla, Dianite, Diopside, Emerald, Eye of the Storm, Fuchsite, Galena (wash hands after use, make essence by indirect method), Graphic Smoky Quartz, Green Jasper, Hanksite, Iron Pyrite, Larimar, Malachite (use as polished stone, make essence by indirect method), Ocean Jasper, Petrified Wood, Quantum Quattro, Rhodozite, Shungite, Siberian Blue Quartz, Spinel, Sulphur in

Quartz, Topaz, Turquoise, Wind Fossil Agate, Zoisite and see Arthritis page 155

> **bladder and intestinal:** Agate Bastnasite, Gaspeite, Honey Calcite, Scheelite
>
> **kidneys:** Brazilianite, Diopside, Jade, Klinoptilolith (wash hands after use, make essence by indirect method), Nunderite, White Chohua Jasper
>
> **joints:** Dianite, Malachite (use as polished stone, make essence by indirect method), Nzuri Moyo, Petrified Wood, Rhodonite, Sulphur in Quartz, Tantalite
>
> **skin:** Chrysotile in Serpentine, Honey Calcite, Riebekite with Sugilite and Bustamite
>
> **urethra:** Scheelite, Yellow Zincite

Influenza: Fluorite, Moss Agate, Quantum Quattro, Que Sera, Shungite. *Chakra:* Higher heart

Insomnia: Ajoite, Ajoite with Shattuckite, Amethyst, Bloodstone, Candle Quartz, Celestite, Charoite, Glendonite, Hematite, Howlite, Khutnohorite, Lapis Lazuli, Lepidolite, Magnetite (Lodestone) (place at head and foot of bed), Moonstone, Mount Shasta Opal, Muscovite, Ocean Jasper, Petrified Wood, Pink Sunstone, Poldarvaarite, Rosophia, Selenite, Shungite, Sodalite, Tektite, Topaz, Zoisite. Place by the bed or under the pillow.

> **disturbed sleep patterns:** Khutnohorite, Ocean Jasper, Owyhee Blue Opal, Petrified Wood, Sodalite
>
> **from geopathic/electromagnetic stress/pollution:**

Black Tourmaline, Chlorite Quartz, Crystal Cap Amethyst, Eye of the Storm, Gabbro, Guinea Fowl Jasper, Herkimer Diamond, Klinoptilolith (wash hands after use, make essence by indirect method), Labradorite, Marble, Ocean Jasper, Orgonite, Red Amethyst, Shieldite, Shungite, Smoky Herkimer Diamond, Smoky Quartz, Sodalite, Spectrolite, Tektite, Thunder Egg. Place around bed and/or around the four corners of the room or house, depending on how strong the stress.

negative environmental influences: Black Tourmaline, Bloodstone, Champagne Aura Quartz, Klinoptilolith (wash hands after use, make essence by indirect method), Lepidolite, Marble, Orgonite, Shungite, Smoky Elestial Quartz, Smoky Quartz, Tantalite, Trummer Jasper, Turquoise. Place around the four corners of the room.

nightmares/night terrors: Dalmatian Stone, Fairy Quartz, Smoky Quartz, Sodalite, Spirit Quartz, Tourmaline, Tremolite. *Chakra:* third eye

overactive mind: Amethyst, Auralite 23, Blue Selenite, Bytownite (Yellow Labradorite), Crystal Cap Amethyst, Rhodozite, Sodalite, Spectrolite. *Chakra:* third eye

stress: Amethyst, Chrysoprase, Eye of the Storm, Lemurian Gold Opal, Riebekite with Sugilite and Bustamite, Rose Quartz, Shungite, Sodalite, Tektite

Unless otherwise directed, place crystal in the environment or on a map, apply over an organ or site of symptom, place on an appropriate chakra, wear as jewellery, or bathe with or use as crystal essence.

and see Stress page 241. *Chakra:* higher heart

Insulin regulation: Astraline, Candle Quartz, Chrysocolla, Malacholla, Maw Sit Sit, Nuummite, Pink Opal, Red Serpentine, Schalenblende, Serpentine in Obsidian, Shungite and see Blood sugar page 162 and Pancreas page 230. *Chakra:* spleen, dantien

> **stabilize:** Ammolite, Septarian. *Chakra:* third eye, crown

Intercellular:

> **blockages:** Fulgarite, Gold in Quartz, Golden Healer Quartz, Plancheite, Pyrite and Sphalerite, Rhodozite, Serpentine in Obsidian

> **structures:** Ajo Blue Calcite, Candle Quartz, Cradle of Life, Gold in Quartz, Golden Healer Quartz, Lemurian Aquitane Calcite, Messina Quartz, Quantum Quattro, Que Sera, Pollucite, Rhodozite, Septarian

Intestinal disorders: Bastnasite, Bismuth, Brown Tourmaline, Cryolite, Gaspeite, Halite, Hanksite, Orange Calcite, Honey Calcite, Scolecite, Septarian. *Chakra:* sacral, dantien

Irritability: Apatite, Fluorapatite, Jade, Pyrite in Magnesite, Rhodonite. *Chakra:* base, sacral, dantien

Irritable bowel syndrome (IBS): Amblygonite, Bastnasite, Calcite, Cryolite, Montebrasite, Pumice, Rosophia, Scolecite, Xenotine. *Chakra:* dantien

Irritant filter: Limestone, Pumice, Rhodochrosite. *Chakra:* dantien

---

Unless otherwise directed, place crystal in the environment or on a map, apply over an organ or site of symptom, place on an appropriate chakra, wear as jewellery, or bathe with or use as crystal essence.

- J -

Jetlag: Preseli Bluestone, Shungite

Joints: Azurite, Calcite, Cat's Eye Quartz, Dioptase, Hematite, Magnetite (Lodestone), Messina Quartz, Petrified Wood, Phantom Calcite, Poldarvaarite, Rhodozite, Rhodonite

    calcified: Calcite, Calcite Fairy Stone, Dinosaur Bone

    flexibility: Bastnasite, Cavansite, Kimberlite, Peach Selenite, Prehnite with Epidote, Selenite Phantom, Strontianite

    inflammation: Hematite, Hematite with Malachite (use as polished stone, make essence by indirect method), Lapis Lazuli, Malachite (use as polished stone, make essence by indirect method), Nzuri Moyo, Peach Selenite, Rhodonite, Rhodozite, Shungite, Sulphur in Quartz, and see Inflammation page 209

    mobilize: Aztee, Calcite Fairy Stone, Fluorite, Nzuri Moyo, Petrified Wood, Prehnite with Epidote, Red Calcite, Strontianite

    pain: Blue Euclase, Cathedral Quartz, Champagne Aura Quartz, Eilat Stone, Flint, Khutnohorite, Nzuri Moyo, Quantum Quattro, Rhodozite, Tantalite

    problems: Amber, Apatite, Fluorite, Lepidolite, Obsidian, Sulphur (use as polished crystallized stone, make essence by indirect method)

Unless otherwise directed, place crystal in the environment or on a map, apply over an organ or site of symptom, place on an appropriate chakra, wear as jewellery, or bathe with or use as crystal essence.

strengthening: Aragonite, Calcite, Clevelandite, Dinosaur Bone, Tantalite

swollen: Malachite (use as polished stone, make essence by indirect method), Nzuri Moyo, Shungite, Trigonic Quartz, and see Inflammation page 209

Unless otherwise directed, place crystal in the environment or on a map, apply over an organ or site of symptom, place on an appropriate chakra, wear as jewellery, or bathe with or use as crystal essence.

- K -

Kidneys: Amber, Aquamarine, Bastnasite, Beryl, Black Moonstone, Bloodstone, Blue Quartz, Brookite, Carnelian, Chohua Jasper, Chrysocolla, Citrine, Conichalcite, Diopside, Fiskenaesset Ruby, Gaspeite, Hematite, Heulandite, Jade, Jadeite, Leopardskin Jasper, Libyan Gold Tektite, Muscovite, Nephrite, Nunderite, Nuummite, Orange Calcite, Prehnite with Epidote, Quantum Quattro, Rhodochrosite, Rose or Smoky Quartz, Rosophia, Septarian, Serpentine, Serpentine in Obsidian, Shungite, Sonora Sunrise, Stromatolite, Tanzanite, Topaz. *Chakra:* dantien, solar plexus. Or tape over kidneys.

> **cleanse:** Atacamite, Bloodstone, Brazilianite, Eye of the Storm (Judy's Jasper), Fire and Ice Quartz, Hematite, Jade, Klinoptilolith (wash hands after use, make essence by indirect method), Nephrite, Nuummite, Opal, Prehnite with Epidote, Red or Yellow Jasper, Rose Quartz
>
> **degeneration:** Honey Calcite, Quantum Quattro, Quartz, Red Jasper, Rosophia, Yellow Jasper
>
> **detoxify:** Amechlorite, Chlorite Quartz, Chohua Jasper, Chrysocolla, Eye of the Storm, Fire and Ice Quartz, Fiskenaesset Ruby, Kambaba Jasper, Klinoptilolith (wash hands after use, make essence by indirect method), Larvikite, Leopardskin Jasper,

---

Unless otherwise directed, place crystal in the environment or on a map, apply over an organ or site of symptom, place on an appropriate chakra, wear as jewellery, or bathe with or use as crystal essence.

Nuummite, Quantum Quattro, Pyrite in Magnesite, Rainbow Covellite, Richterite, Seraphinite, Shungite, Smoky Quartz, Smoky Quartz with Aegerine

fortify: Grossular Garnet, Heulandite, Quartz

infection: Citrine, Yellow Zincite

regulating: Carnelian, Muscovite

stimulating: Ruby, Rhodochrosite

stones: Jasper, Magnesite, Rhyolite

underactive: Fire Opal, Prehnite, Rhodochrosite, Ruby

Knees: Aragonite, Azurite, Blue Lace Agate, Cathedral Quartz, Dinosaur Bone

Unless otherwise directed, place crystal in the environment or on a map, apply over an organ or site of symptom, place on an appropriate chakra, wear as jewellery, or bathe with or use as crystal essence.

- L -

Legs: Ametrine, Aquamarine, Bloodstone, Blue Tiger's Eye, Carnelian, Garnet, Hawk's Eye, Jasper, Pietersite, Red Tiger's Eye, Ruby, Smoky Quartz, Tourmaline. *Chakra:* base, sacral

Lethargy: Ametrine, Carnelian, Red Tiger's Eye, Ruby, Tourmaline. *Chakra:* base, sacral

Leukaemia: Alexandrite, Bloodstone, Uvarovite Garnet

Life force, increase: Aquamarine, Triplite. *Chakra:* higher heart. Wear continuously.

Liver: Amber, Amethyst, Aquamarine, Azurite with Malachite (use as polished stone, make essence by indirect method), Beryl, Black Moonstone, Bloodstone, Blue Holly Agate, Brookite, Carnelian, Charoite, Chrysoprase, Cinnabar in Jasper, Citrine, Danburite, Eilat Stone, Emerald, Empowerite, Epidote, Fluorite, Gaspeite, Gold Calcite, Golden Danburite, Guinea Fowl Jasper, Heulandite, Hiddenite, Huebnerite, Labradorite, Lazulite, Lepidocrosite, Limonite, Poppy Jasper, Orange River Quartz, Pietersite, Red Amethyst, Red Jasper, Rhodonite, Rose Quartz, Ruby, Shungite, Tiger's Eye, Topaz, Tugtupite, Yellow Fluorite, Yellow Jasper, Yellow Labradorite. *Chakra:* dantien

> **blockages:** Bastnasite, Fulgarite, Gaspeite, Holly Agate, Orange Kyanite, Poppy Jasper, Red Jasper, Red Tourmaline, Rhodozite, Thunder Egg

---

Unless otherwise directed, place crystal in the environment or on a map, apply over an organ or site of symptom, place on an appropriate chakra, wear as jewellery, or bathe with or use as crystal essence.

blood flow: Mookaite Jasper

cleanse: Charoite, Crystal Cap Amethyst, Gaspeite, Klinoptilolith (wash hands after use, make essence by indirect method), Peridot, Ruby

depletion: Holly Agate, Macedonian Opal, Tugtupite

detoxifying: Amechlorite, Bastnasite, Biotite, Chlorite Quartz, Eye of the Storm, Gaspeite, Kambaba Jasper, Klinoptilolith (wash hands after use, make essence by indirect method), Larvikite, Malachite (use as polished stone, make essence by indirect method), Mtrolite, Pyrite in Magnesite, Rainbow Covellite, Richterite, Seraphinite, Shungite, Smoky Quartz with Aegerine, Thunder Egg

stimulate: Amethyst, Azurite, Emerald, Poppy Jasper, Schalenblende, Silver Leaf Jasper, Tantalite, Thunder Egg, Tugtupite, Zircon

Lungs: Adamite, Amber, Amethyst, Ammolite, Andean Blue Opal, Atlantasite, Aventurine, Beryl, Blue Aragonite, Blue Quartz, Botswana Agate, Bustamite, Cacoxenite, Catlinite, Charoite, Chrysocolla, Diopside, Dioptase, Emerald, Fluorapatite, Fluorite, Graphic Smoky Quartz (Zebra Stone), Greenlandite, Hiddenite, Kambaba Jasper, Kunzite, Lapis Lazuli, Morganite, Peridot, Petalite, Petrified Wood, Pink Tourmaline, Prehnite, Prehnite with Epidote, Pyrite in Quartz, Quantum Quattro, Rhodochrosite, Rose Quartz, Sardonyx, Scheelite, Scolecite, Serpentine, Serpentine in Obsidian, Smoky

Amethyst, Sodalite, Sonora Sunrise, Stromatolite, Tremolite, Turquoise, Valentinite and Stibnite, Watermelon Tourmaline. *Chakra:* dantien, higher heart

> **congested:** Kambaba Jasper, Moss Agate, Quantum Quattro, Shungite, Stromatolite, Vanadinite (wash hands after use, make essence by indirect method)

> **difficulty in breathing:** Anthrophyllite, Apophyllite, Chrysocolla, Green Siberian Quartz, Kambaba Jasper, Quantum Quattro, Riebekite with Sugilite and Bustamite, Stromatolite, Tremolite and see Breathlessness page 219

> **fluid in:** Amber, Diamond, Hackmanite, Halite, Hanksite, Ocean Jasper, Scheelite, Smoky Amethyst, Yellow Sapphire, Zircon

Lupus: Chinese Red Quartz, Eudialyte

Lymph: Bloodstone, Chalcedony, Chrysoprase, Moonstone, Shungite, Trigonic Quartz

Lymphatic system: Agate, Anglesite, Bastnasite, Blue Chalcedony, Chlorite Quartz, Eye of the Storm (Judy's Jasper), Graphic Smoky Quartz, Hackmanite, Lazulite, Moonstone, Moss Agate, Ocean Blue Jasper, Scheelite, Shungite, Tourmaline, Trigonic Quartz, Zebra Stone. *Chakra:* dantien, higher heart

> **cleansing:** Agate, Bastnasite, Chlorite Quartz, Crystal Cap Amethyst, Feather Pyrite, Ocean Jasper, Rose Quartz, Shungite, Sodalite, Sugilite, Yellow Apatite

> **infections:** Blue Lace Agate, Shungite

stimulating: Bloodstone, Blue Chalcedony, Ocean Jasper, Oligocrase

swellings: Agrellite, Anandalite™, Blue Euclase, Crystal Cap Amethyst, Jet

Unless otherwise directed, place crystal in the environment or on a map, apply over an organ or site of symptom, place on an appropriate chakra, wear as jewellery, or bathe with or use as crystal essence.

- M -

ME: Ametrine, Bismuth, Chinese Red Quartz, Chrysolite in Serpentine, Eye of the Storm, Petrified Wood, Quantum Quattro, Que Sera, Ruby, Shungite, Tourmaline. *Chakra:* dantien

Memory, improve: Amber, Amethyst, Barite, Coprolite, Emerald, Fluorite, Hematoid Calcite, Herderite, Klinoptilolith (wash hands after use, make essence by indirect method), Marcasite, Moss Agate, Opal, Phantom Calcite, Pyrite and Sphalerite, Pyrolusite, Rhodonite, Unakite, Vivianite. *Chakra:* third eye, crown

Menderes disease: Ammolite, Dioptase. Tape behind affected ear.

Mental harmony: Auralite 23, Bytownite (Yellow Labradorite), Fluorite. *Chakra:* third eye

Metabolic:

> **imbalances:** Amazonite, Amechlorite, Azurite with Malachite and Chrysocolla (use as polished stone, make essence by indirect method), Blue Opal, Bornite, Champagne Aura Quartz, Chrysocolla, Diamond, Galaxyite, Garnet, Golden Azeztulite, Golden Danburite, Golden Herkimer, Hackmanite, Healer's Gold, Herkimer Diamond, Khutnohorite, Labradorite, Lemurian Jade, Mangano Vesuvianite, Peridot, Quantum Quattro, Que Sera, Shungite, Sonora Sunrise, Tantalite, Tanzine Aura Quartz, Tugtupite,

Unless otherwise directed, place crystal in the environment or on a map, apply over an organ or site of symptom, place on an appropriate chakra, wear as jewellery, or bathe with or use as crystal essence.

Watermelon Tourmaline, Winchite. *Chakra:* dantien, third eye

stimulate processes: Apatite, Blue Tiger's Eye, Garnet, Hawk's Eye, Red Carnelian, Smoky Amethyst, Tugtupite. *Chakra:* brow and dantien

syndrome: Amechlorite, Anandalite, Andara Glass, Galaxyite, Klinoptilolith (wash hands after use, make essence by indirect method), Quantum Quattro, Que Sera, Richterite, Scheelite, Shungite, Tanzine Aura Quartz, Winchite

system: Amechlorite, Amethyst, Bloodstone, Carnelian, Champagne Aura Quartz, Hackmanite, Labradorite, Piemontite, Smoky Amethyst, Smoky Quartz with Aegerine, Sodalite, Tantalite, Winchite

Metabolism: Amazonite, Amechlorite, Ametrine, Bloodstone, Chrysoprase, Dendritic Agate, Fossilised Wood, Galaxyite, Garnet, Garnet in Pyroxene, Klinoptilolith (wash hands after use, make essence by indirect method), Labradorite, Piemontite, Quantum Quattro, Que Sera, Ruby, Serpentine, Shungite, Sodalite, Tourmaline, Tree Agate, Turquoise, Winchite

stimulate: Amethyst, Garnet, Pyrolusite, Sodalite. *Chakra:* higher heart

Microwaves: Amazonite, Amethyst, Black Moonstone, Black Tourmaline, Chlorite Quartz, Fluorite, Gabbro, Germanium, Granite, Graphic Smoky Quartz, Hematite, Herkimer Diamond, Klinoptilolith (wash hands after use, make essence by indirect method), Malachite (use as polished stone, make essence by indirect method), Orgonite, Reinerite, Shieldite, Shungite, Smoky Elestial Quartz, Smoky Quartz, Sodalite, Sphalerite, Tourmalinated Quartz, Tourmaline, Yellow Kunzite, Zeolite. Place around site or between you and the site.

Migraine: Amethyst, Aventurine, Azurite, Cathedral Quartz, Dioptase, Iolite, Jet, Lapis Lazuli, Magnesite, Pearl, Rhodochrosite, Rose Quartz, Sodalite, Sugilite, Topaz. *Chakra:* brow, crown, past life

Mood swings: Amazonite, Kunzite, Serpentine, Turquoise

Motor Dysfunction: Danburite, Kyanite, Sugilite

Muscles: Bismuth, Black Kyanite, Cat's Eye Quartz, Hematite, Jadeite, Nzuri Moyo, Petrified Wood, Phlogopite, Rhodonite, Scheelite, Titanite (Sphene)

cramps: Apache Tear, Bastnasite, Cat's Eye Quartz, Celestite, Infinite Stone, Larimar, Magnesite, Magnetite (Lodestone), Orange Moss Agate, Quantum Quattro, Serpentine in Obsidian, Smithsonite, Strontianite and see page 185

disorders: Diopside, Kyanite, Peridot, Petalite, Rosophia

dystrophy: Rosophia, Scolecite and Natrolite

flexibility/pain: Aegerine, Blue Euclase, Cathedral Quartz, Eilat Stone, Flint, Rhodozite, Wind Fossil Agate

Unless otherwise directed, place crystal in the environment or on a map, apply over an organ or site of symptom, place on an appropriate chakra, wear as jewellery, or bathe with or use as crystal essence.

spasm: Amazonite, Apache Tear, Azurite with Malachite (use as polished stone, make essence by indirect method), Bornite, Chrysocolla, Diopside, Fuchsite, Magnetite (Lodestone), Malacholla, Petalite, Phlogopite, Pyrite in Magnesite, Red Tourmaline, Strontianite and see Spasms page 240

strengthen: Aegerine, Apatite, Bismuth, Bustamite, Fluorite, Jadeite, Peridot, Tourmaline

swelling: Anandalite™, Andean Blue Opal, Blue Euclase, Brochantite

tension: Basalt, Blue Aragonite, Blue Euclase, Champagne Aura Quartz

tissue: Aventurine, Danburite, Desert Rose, Khutnohorite, Magnetite (Lodestone), Phlogopite, Sonora Sunrise

tone: Fluorite, Peridot, Tourmaline

weak: Tiger Iron, Rhyolite

Muscular-skeletal system inflexibility: Fuchsite, Jade, Magnesite, Coprolite, Cumberlandite, Kimberlite, Limonite, Quantum Quattro, Rosophia, Steatite, Stromatolite

---

Unless otherwise directed, place crystal in the environment or on a map, apply over an organ or site of symptom, place on an appropriate chakra, wear as jewellery, or bathe with or use as crystal essence.

- N -

Nausea: Brown Agate, Dioptase, Emerald, Fuchsite, Green Jasper, Red Aventurine, Sapphire

Negative:

    energy dispel: Amber, Amethyst, Black Tourmaline, Heulandite, Lapis Lazuli, Orgonite, Pollucite, Scolecite, Shungite, Smoky Quartz, Snowflake Obsidian, Sodalite, Stilbite, Thomsonite, and see Detoxification page 188

    ions, increase: Amethyst, Angel's Wing Calcite, Bismuth, Germanium, Heulandite, Jasper, Klinoptilolith (wash hands after use, make essence by indirect method), Lepidolite, Orgonite, Pollucite, Quartz, Renierite, Scolecite, Shungite, Sphalerite, Stilbite, Thomsonite, Tourmaline

Nerves: Bronzite, Cat's Eye Quartz, Cryolite, Dalmatian Stone, Golden Coracalcite, Merlinite, Natrolite, Nuummite, Phlogopite, Scheelite, Scolecite, Smoky Amethyst, Stichtite, Tanzanite

    calming: Eudialyte, Jamesonite

    endings: Guinea Fowl Jasper, Tinguaite

    motor: Bustamite, Cat's Eye Quartz

    optic: see Eyes page xx

    pain relief: Blue Euclase, Flint, Nuummite, Rhodozite, Wind Fossil Agate

    regenerating: Natrolite with Scolecite

spinal: Tinguaite

strengthen: Banded Agate, Drusy Quartz on Sphalerite, Mystic Topaz, Nuummite

Nervous:

autonomic system: Anglesite, Aventurine, Barite, Datolite, Dendritic Chalcedony, Golden Coracalcite, Kambaba Jasper, Merlinite, Phantom Calcite, Stichtite, Stromatolite, White Heulandite. *Chakra:* dantien

disorders: Natrolite with Scolecite

exhaustion: Cinnabar in Jasper, Eudialyte

stress: Auralite 23, Eudialyte, Eye of the Storm, Larvikite, Merlinite, Riebekite with Sugilite and Bustamite, Shungite

sympathetic: Cumberlandite. *Chakra:* dantien and see page 242

system: Aegerine, Alexandrite, Anglesite, Astrophyllite, Azeztulite with Morganite, Banded Agate, Datolite, Dendritic Chalcedony, Epidote, Eudialyte, Greenlandite, Kakortokite, Larvikite, Merlinite, Natrolite, Petrified Wood, Prehnite with Epidote, Scolecite, Stichtite, Stichtite and Serpentine, Tremolite, White Heulandite

tension: Larvikite, Merlinite

Neural:

pathways: Golden Coracalcite, Larvikite, Merlinite, Mystic Merlinite, Natrolite, Phantom Calcite, Scolecite, Stichtite, Tree Agate

---

Unless otherwise directed, place crystal in the environment or on a map, apply over an organ or site of symptom, place on an appropriate chakra, wear as jewellery, or bathe with or use as crystal essence.

transmission: Anglesite, Larvikite, Natrolite, Scolecite, Tremolite

Neurological tissue: Alexandrite, Golden Coracalcite, Natrolite, Phlogopite, Scolecite and see Nerves above

Neurotransmitters: Anglesite, Crystal Cap Amethyst, Golden Coracalcite, Kambaba Jasper, Khutnohorite, Ocean Blue Jasper, Phantom Calcite, Que Sera, Scolecite, Shungite, Sodalite, Stromatolite, Tremolite. *Chakra:* alta major (base of skull)

Nightmares/night terrors: Amethyst, Celestite, Chrysoprase, Dalmatian Stone, Diaspore, Hematite, Jet, Mangano Calcite, Pearl Spa Dolomite, Prehnite, Rose Quartz, Ruby, Spirit Quartz, Tremolite, Turquoise, Smoky Quartz, Sodalite. Place under the pillow or around the bed.

Nuclear sites, transmute radiation effects: Amber, Aventurine, Boron, Chlorite Quartz, Colemanite, Covellite, Galena (wash hands after use, make essence by indirect method), Graphic Smoky Quartz, Hackmanite, Kernite, Larimar, Lepidolite, Libyan Gold Tektite, Malachite (use as polished stone, make essence by indirect method), Malacholla, Mica, Morion, Orgonite, Rainbow Covellite, Smoky Elestial Quartz, Smoky Quartz, Shungite, Sodalite, Tantalite, Tektite, Torbernite (under supervision), Velvet Malachite (wash hands after use, make essence by indirect method). Place stones around site or between you and the source.

Unless otherwise directed, place crystal in the environment or on a map, apply over an organ or site of symptom, place on an appropriate chakra, wear as jewellery, or bathe with or use as crystal essence.

Nutrient malabsorption: Blue Moonstone, Candle Quartz, Fluorite, Idocrase, Moonstone, Pietersite, Serpentine, Turquoise. *Chakra:* solar plexus

- O -

Obesity: Black Onyx, Diamond, Moonstone, Tourmaline, Zircon

Oversensitive personality: Bastnasite, Hackmanite

Oversensitivity to:

    cold: Barite

    pressure: Avalonite

    temperature changes: Barite, Dinosaur Bone, Luxullianite

    weather: Avalonite, Barite, Golden Pietersite

Oxygen, malabsorption: Azotic Topaz, Banded Agate, Chinese Red Quartz, Goethite, Kambaba Jasper, Merlinite, Molybdenite, Pyrite in Magnesite, Pyrite in Quartz, Reinerite, Sonora Sunrise, Stromatolite. *Chakra:* dantien. Or place over heart and lungs.

- P -

Pain relief: Amber, Amethyst, Aragonite, Boji Stones, Cathedral Quartz, Celestite, Dendritic Agate, Fluorite, Hematite, Infinite Stone, Lapis Lazuli, Larimar, Magnetite (Lodestone), Mahogany Obsidian, Malachite (use as polished stone, make essence by indirect method), Quartz, Rose Quartz, Seraphinite, Smoky Quartz, Sugilite, Tourmaline

Palpitations: Amber, Danburite, Dumortierite, Eye of the Storm, Garnet, Honey Calcite, Rose Quartz, Tugtupite. *Chakra:* dantien and heart

Pancreas: Amber, Astraline, Bloodstone, Blue Lace Agate, Brochantite, Bustamite, Carnelian, Charoite, Chinese Chromium Quartz, Chrysocolla, Citrine, Green Calcite, Huebnerite, Jasper, Leopardskin Jasper, Malachite (use as polished stone, make essence by indirect method), Maw Sit Sit, Moonstone, Pink Opal, Pink Tourmaline, Quantum Quattro, Red Tourmaline, Richterite, Schalenblende, Septarian, Serpentine in Obsidian, Shungite, Smoky Quartz, Tanzine Aura Quartz, Topaz, Tugtupite. *Chakra:* spleen, dantien

Pancreatic secretions: Astraline, Bustamite, Malachite (use as polished stone, make essence by indirect method), Muscovite. *Chakra:* spleen, solar plexus, base and see Blood sugar page 162

Panic attacks: Amethyst, Blue-green Smithsonite,

Dumortierite, Eye of the Storm, Girasol, Green Phantom Quartz, Green Tourmaline, Kunzite, Serpentine in Obsidian, Tremolite, Turquoise. *Chakra:* heart, higher heart, solar plexus. Keep in pocket and hold when required.

Parathyroid: Blue Siberian Quartz, Cacoxenite, Champagne Aura Quartz, Chrysotile, Chrysotile in Serpentine, Cumberlandite, Kyanite, Leopardskin Jasper, Malachite (use as polished stone, make essence by indirect method), Richterite, Tanzine Aura Quartz. *Chakra:* throat

Parkinson's disease: Anthrophyllite, Black Moonstone, Diaspore, Eudialyte, Kambaba Jasper, Nuummite, Owyhee Blue Opal, Stichtite, Stichtite and Serpentine, Stromatolite. *Chakra:* dantien

Physical:

body, discomfort at being in: Candle Quartz, Empowerite, Eye of the Storm, Larvikite, Pearl Spa Dolomite, Phenacite, Picasso Jasper, Strontianite, Vanadinite (wash hands after use, make essence by indirect method). *Chakra:* earth star, base, dantien, soma

endurance, improve: Poppy Jasper, Schalenblende, Sodalite, Triplite. *Chakra:* earth star, base, dantien

exhaustion: Eye of the Storm, Mariposite, Poppy Jasper, Purpurite, Strawberry Lemurian (Red Lemurian Seed Crystal), Vanadinite (wash hands after use, make essence by indirect method). *Chakra:* earth star, base, dantien

pleasure, share: Poppy Jasper. *Chakra:* earth star, base

weakness: Diopside, Schalenblende, Sedona Stone. *Chakra:* dantien

well-being: Cloudy Quartz, Golden Healer Quartz, Guardian Stone, Keyiapo, Quantum Quattro, Que Sera, Schalenblende, Sedona Stone, Shungite. *Chakra:* earth star, base, dantien

Pineal gland: Amethyst, Blue Moonstone, Champagne Aura Quartz, Fire and Ice Quartz, Fluorapatite, Gem Rhodonite, Moonstone, Opal, Petalite, Preseli Bluestone, Quartz, Richterite, Ruby, Tanzanite, Tanzine Aura Quartz, Tremolite Sodalite, Yellow Labradorite. *Chakra:* third eye

Pituitary gland: Apatite, Chalcopyrite, Champagne Aura Quartz, Charoite, Elbaite, Fire and Ice Quartz, Labradorite, Rhodonite, Sugilite, Tanzine Aura Quartz. *Chakra:* third eye

Pneumonia: Diamond, Fluorite, Shungite

Polarization (re-align to earth's magnetic field): Eye of the Storm, Labradorite, Preseli Bluestone

Pollutants, anti: Amazonite, Amber, Aventurine, Black Tourmaline, Brown Jasper, Chlorite Quartz, Malachite (use as polished stone, make essence by indirect method), Orgonite, Purple Tourmaline, Quantum Quattro, Shieldite, Shungite, Sodalite, Turquoise. *Chakra:* earth star. Place stones in environment to absorb.

Psoriasis: Blue Lace Agate, Labradorite, Snakeskin Agate and see Ski page 238. Bathe in crystal essence and apply stone to site.

Pulse, irregular: Agate, Charoite. Wear over heart.

Unless otherwise directed, place crystal in the environment or on a map, apply over an organ or site of symptom, place on an appropriate chakra, wear as jewellery, or bathe with or use as crystal essence.

- Q -

Qi: *Chakra:* sacral, dantien

    depleted: Ammolite, Budd Stone (African Jade), Chalcopyrite, Granite, Judy's Jasper, Kyanite, Magnetite (Lodestone), Poppy Jasper, Que Sera, Ruby in Granite, Rhodozite, Sonora Sunrise, Violane, Witches Finger, Zincite

    transmit: Feather Pyrite, Green Ridge Quartz, Que Sera, Rhodozite, Terraluminite

Radiation, counteract: Aventurine, Black Tourmaline, Boron, Chlorite Quartz, Colemanite, Covellite, Galena (wash hands after use, make essence by indirect method), Graphic Smoky Quartz, Hackmanite, Jasper, Kernite, Klinoptilolith (wash hands after use, make essence by indirect method), Kunzite, Malachite (use as polished stone, make essence by indirect method), Morion, Orgonite, Ouro Verde, Quartz, Rainbow Covellite, Reinerite, Smoky Elestial Quartz, Smoky Quartz, Sodalite, Tantalite, Tektite, Torbernite, Uranophane, Velvet Malachite (use as polished stone, make essence by indirect method), Yellow Kunzite. *Chakra:* earth star, base. Place stones around source.

Radioactivity: Annabergite, Boron, Chlorite Quartz, Colemanite, Galena (wash hands after use, make essence by indirect method), Herkimer Diamond, Kernite, Kunzite, Malachite (use as polished stone, make essence by indirect method), Orgonite, Reinerite. Place stones around source or wear continuously.

Radon gas: Boron, Chlorite Quartz, Covellite, Danburite, Diaspore, Eye of the Storm (rough form), Graphic Smoky Quartz, Herkimer Diamond, Klinoptilolith (wash hands after use, make essence by indirect method), Libyan Gold Tektite, Malachite (use as polished stone, make essence by indirect method), Morion Quartz, Nifontovite, Ouro

Verde, Shungite, Smoky Elestial Quartz, Smoky Quartz, Sodalite, Tektite, Torbernite, Yellow Kunzite. Place stones around source.

Relaxation: Amethyst, Aventurine, Blue Calcite, Dioptase, Fire Agate, Fuchsite, Golden Calcite, Jasper, Magnesite, Peridot, Rhodonite, Smoky Quartz

Repair, assist body to: Aegerine, Bixbite, Brandenberg Amethyst, Celestial Quartz, Molybdenite, Quantum Quattro, Rutile with Hematite, Shungite, Zoisite. *Chakra:* dantien

Reproductive system: Beryllonite, Black Kyanite, Calcite Fairy Stone, Fire and Ice Quartz, Lepidocrosite, Menalite, Voegesite, Xenotine. *Chakra:* base, sacral, dantien

>   **fallopian tubes:** Menalite, Schalenblende. *Chakra:* sacral

>   **female:** Black Moonstone, Fire and Ice Quartz, Menalite, Schalenblende, Tangerose. *Chakra:* sacral, base

>   **inflammation:** Blue Euclase, Dendritic Chalcedony, Hanksite, Kundalini Quartz, Rhodozite, Sulphur in Quartz

>   **male:** Calcite Fairy Stone, Schalenblende, Shiva Lingam

>   **ovaries:** Menalite, Schalenblende

>   **testicles:** Alexandrite, Schalenblende. *Chakra:* base

Respiratory system: Blue Aragonite, Cacoxenite, Halite, Kambaba Jasper, Merlinite, Prophecy Stone, Pyrite in

Quartz, Quantum Quattro, Richterite, Riebekite with Sugilite and Bustamite, Smoky Amethyst, Snakeskin Pyrite, Stromatolite, Tremolite. *Chakra:* dantien, higher heart

problems: Cacoxenite, Kambaba Jasper, Riebekite with Sugilite and Bustamite, Smoky Amethyst, Stromatolite, Tremolite

Unless otherwise directed, place crystal in the environment or on a map, apply over an organ or site of symptom, place on an appropriate chakra, wear as jewellery, or bathe with or use as crystal essence.

- S -

Seasonal affective disorder: Sunstone, Sunshine Aura Quartz, Topaz, Triplite. Wear continuously.

Senile dementia: Anthrophyllite, Chalcedony, Rose Quartz, Stichtite and Serpentine. *Chakra:* third eye. Base of skull or wear continuously.

Senior moments: Barite, Blue or Black Moonstone, Hematoid Calcite, Herderite, Marcasite, Vivianite. *Chakra:* third eye. Or place at base of skull.

Shield yourself: Black Tourmaline, Healer's Gold, Nuummite, Polychrome Jasper, Pyrite, Shieldite, Shungite, Smoky Quartz. *Chakra:* higher heart

Sick building syndrome: Black Tourmaline, Chlorite Quartz, Covellite, Galena (wash hands after use, make essence by indirect method), Graphic Smoky Quartz, Hackmanite, Lepidolite, Marble, Morion, Orgonite, Preseli Bluestone, Quartz, Selenite, Shieldite, Shungite, Smoky Elestial Quartz, Smoky Quartz, Sodalite, Trummer Jasper. Place around building, in zigzag in room (see page 122), or wear constantly.

Skin: Agate, Amethyst, Aventurine, Azurite, Brown Jasper, Bustamite, Chohua Jasper, Eisenkiesel, Epidote, Ethiopian Opal, Green Jasper, Galena (wash hands after use, make essence by indirect method), Guinea Fowl Jasper, Halite, Hanksite, Honey Calcite, Kieseltuff, Klinoptilolith (wash hands after use, make essence by

Unless otherwise directed, place crystal in the environment or on a map, apply over an organ or site of symptom, place on an appropriate chakra, wear as jewellery, or bathe with or use as crystal essence.

indirect method), Pearl Spa Dolomite, Phosphosiderite, Prehnite with Epidote, Rose Quartz, Riebekite with Sugilite and Bustamite, Snakeskin Agate, Stichtite, Sulphur (use as polished crystallized stone, make essence by indirect method), Topaz, Titanite (Sphene). *Chakra:* higher heart. Or place over site.

cancer: Emerald, Fluorapatite, Klinoptilolith (wash hands after use, make essence by indirect method) (place over site) and see Cancer page 167

detoxify: Aegerine, Amechlorite, Chlorite Quartz, Eye of the Storm, Graphic Smoky Quartz, Jamesonite, Larvikite, Lepidolite, Pyrite in Magnesite, Richterite, Seraphinite, Shungite, Smoky Elestial Quartz, Smoky Quartz with Aegerine, Rainbow Covellite, Shungite, Stichtite

disorders: Agate, Brown and Green Jasper, Calcite, Green Aventurine, Erythrite, Leopardskin Jasper, Chrysoprase, Fluorite, Pearl, Rhyolite, Rose Quartz, Rhodochrosite, Smithsonite, Snowflake Obsidian, Spirit Quartz, Sulphur, Zircon (use as polished crystallized stone, make essence by indirect method)

elasticity: Epidote, Flint, Novaculite, Stichtite

encrustations: Drusy Golden Healer, Faden Quartz, Prophecy Stone, Wind Fossil Agate

growths: Chlorite, Kieseltuff, Wind Fossil Agate

infections: Klinoptilolith (wash hands after use, make essence by indirect method), Libyan Glass, Moss

Agate, Pargasite, Pentagonite, Phosphosiderite, Shungite, Snakeskin Agate, Sulphur (use as polished crystallized stone, make essence by indirect method), Tektite (bathe in crystal water)

inflammation: Chrysotile in Serpentine, Guinea Fowl Jasper, Rhodozite, Sulphur in Quartz

Sleep: see Insomnia page 210

Spasms: Amazonite, Aragonite, Azurite, Carnelian, Magnesite, Electric-blue Obsidian, Ruby

Spleen: Aegerine, Amber, Apple Aura Quartz, Aquamarine, Aventurine, Azurite, Black Moonstone, Bloodstone, Blue Quartz, Brochantite, Bustamite, Chalcedony, Cinnabar in Jasper, Citrine, Fluorite, Gaspeite, Green Obsidian, Guinea Fowl Jasper, Jade, Marcasite, Mookaite Jasper, Nunderite, Orange River Quartz, Peridot, Red Obsidian, Red Tourmaline, Ruby, Septarian, Sunstone, Yellow Labradorite, Wulfenite, Zircon. *Chakra:* spleen

   blood flow: Mookaite Jasper

   deterioration: Mookaite Jasper, Prasiolite

   detoxifying: Amechlorite, Banded Agate, Chlorite Quartz, Eye of the Storm, Jamesonite, Larvikite, Pyrite in Magnesite, Rainbow Covellite, Richterite, Seraphinite, Shungite, Smoky Quartz with Aegerine

   protection: Aventurine, Gaspeite, Green Aventurine, Jade, Nunderite, Tugtupite

Stagnant energy, disperse: Black Tourmaline, Calcite,

Chrome Diopside, Clear Topaz, Eye of the Storm, Garnet in Quartz, Orgonite, Poppy Jasper, Quartz, Ruby Lavender Quartz, Sedona Stone, Shaman Quartz, Shungite, Smoky Quartz, Spirit Quartz, Tantalite and see Negative energy page 225. *Chakra:* base, dantien

Stomach: Amber, Amblygonite, Amethyst, Aquamarine, Beryl, Bismuth, Black Moonstone, Bytownite, Carnelian, Chrysocolla, Cryolite, Fire Agate, Green Fluorite, Jade, Jadeite, Mookaite Jasper, Paraiba Tourmaline, Pearl, Prasiolite, Serpentine, Serpentine in Obsidian, Shungite, Snakeskin Agate, Snowflake Obsidian, Stibnite, Turritella Agate, Tugtupite, Yellow Jasper, Yellow Labradorite. *Chakra:* solar plexus

> **cramps:** Bastnasite, Cat's Eye Quartz, Magnesite, Orange Moss Agate, Serpentine in Obsidian, Zircon
>
> **pains:** Jet, Lapis Lazuli
>
> **problems as a result of stress:** Amechlorite, Barite, Bird's Eye Jasper, Chrysoprase, Eisenkiesel, Eye of the Storm, Marble, Riebekite with Sugilite and Bustamite, Shungite
>
> **ulcer:** Agate, Blue Siberian Quartz, Hemimorphite, Moonstone, Pearl, Quartz, Tiger's Eye

Stress: Amber, Amethyst, Aquamarine, Aventurine, Beryl, Brandenberg Amethyst, Charoite, Dioptase, Eye of the Storm, Galaxyite, Golden Healer Quartz, Graphic Smoky Quartz, Green Aventurine, Herkimer Diamond, Jade, Jasper, Labradorite, Lapis Lazuli, Magnetite,

Marble, Petalite, Quantum Quattro, Que Sera, Rhodonite, Richterite, Rose Quartz, Serpentine, Shungite, Siberian Quartz, Smoky Quartz, Sodalite, Vera Cruz Amethyst

Supra-adrenals: Amber, Amethyst, Aquamarine, Axinite, Beryl, Cacoxenite, Charoite, Dioptase, Epidote, Eye of the Storm, Gaspeite, Green Aventurine, Herkimer Diamond, Jasper, Labradorite, Lapis Lazuli, Magnetite (Lodestone), Nunderite, Petalite, Picrolite, Rhodonite, Richterite, Rose Quartz, Siberian Quartz. *Chakra:* dantien. Or tape over kidneys.

Sympathetic nervous system: Cumberlandite, Golden Healer Quartz

- T -

Tachycardia: Amber, Danburite, Garnet, Rose Quartz, Tugtupite

T-cells: Bloodstone, Diaspore (Zultanite), Dioptase, Klinoptilolith (wash hands after use, make essence by indirect method), Quantum Quattro, Que Sera, Richterite, Rosophia, Shungite, Tangerine Sun Aura Quartz, Tangerose, and see Immune system page 208. *Chakra:* higher heart

    encourage production: Diaspore, Golden Healer Quartz, Klinoptilolith (wash hands after use, make essence by indirect method), Shungite, Tangerose

Thymus: Amethyst, Andean Opal, Angelite, Aqua Aura, Aventurine, Bloodstone, Blue or Green Tourmaline, Blue Halite, Chrysotile, Citrine, Diaspore, Dioptase, Eilat Stone, Hiddenite, Indicolite Quartz, Jadeite, Klinoptilolith (wash hands after use, make essence by indirect method), Lapis Lazuli, Peridot, Prehnite with Epidote, Quantum Quattro, Quartz, Que Sera, Richterite, Rose Quartz, Septarian, Shaman Quartz, Stromatolite, Thomsonite, Tremolite. *Chakra:* higher heart

    underactive: Aqua Aura Quartz, Eilat Stone, Hiddenite, Lapis Lazuli, Peridot, Quantum Quattro, Que Sera, Smithsonite

Thyroid: Amber, Aqua Aura, Aquamarine, Azurite, Beryl, Blue Halite, Blue Tourmaline, Candle Quartz,

Celestite, Champagne Aura Quartz, Citrine, Cryolite, Cumberlandite, Eilat Stone, Idocrase, Indicolite Quartz, Kyanite, Lapis Lazuli, Lavender Aura Quartz, Lazulite, Leopardskin Serpentine, Paraiba Tourmaline, Prehnite with Epidote, Quantum Quattro, Rhodonite, Richterite, Rutilated Quartz, Sapphire, Sodalite, Turquoise, Vanadinite (wash hands after use, make essence by indirect method). *Chakra:* throat

balance: Aquamarine, Cacoxenite, Richterite

deficiencies: Angelite, Blue Lace Agate, Citrine, Harlequin Quartz, Kyanite, Lapis Lazuli, Tanzine Aura Quartz

regulate: Lapis Lazuli, Rhodonite, Richterite, Tanzine Aura Quartz

stimulate: Rhodonite, Rutilated Quartz, Tanzine Aura Quartz. *Chakra:* throat

Tiredness, chronic: Amethyst, Bismuth, Carnelian, Chlorite Quartz, Cinnabar Jasper, Eudialyte, Eye of the Storm, Fire Agate, Fire Obsidian, Golden Healer Quartz, Hematite, Iron Pyrite, Poppy Jasper, Purpurite, Quantum Quattro, Que Sera, Red Jasper, Rose Quartz, Ruby, Ruby in Fuchsite, Tiger Iron, Triplite, and see Fatigue page 199. *Chakra*: base, dantien

Tissue:

connective: Desert Rose, Greenlandite, Piemontite, Prehnite with Epidote

degeneration: Alexandrite, Amber Eilat Stone,

Tantalite

detoxify: Amechlorite, Chlorite Quartz, Eye of the Storm, Fairy Quartz, Green Ridge Quartz, Jamesonite, Larvikite, Phlogopite, Pyrite in Magnesite, Rainbow Covellite, Richterite, Seraphinite, Shungite, Smoky Amethyst, Smoky Quartz with Aegerine, Tantalite

hardened: Prehnite with Epidote, Pumice

regeneration: Alexandrite, Amber, Eilat Stone, Flint, Leopardskin Jasper, Nuummite, Tantalite

repair: Alexandrite, Diaspore (Zultanite), Eilat Stone, Eisenkiesel, Flint, Greenlandite, Khutnohorite, Piemontite, Tantalite

Toxic earth meridians: Amber, Chlorite Quartz, Granite, Graphic Smoky Quartz, Kambaba Jasper, Marble, Mohawkite (use as polished stone, make essence by indirect method), Orgonite, Preseli Bluestone, Quartz, Shieldite, Shungite, Smoky Elestial Quartz, Snakeskin Pyrite, Sodalite, Valentinite and Stibnite

Toxicity: Amber, Arsenopyrite, Champagne Aura Quartz, Chlorite Quartz, Green Jasper, Klinoptilolith (wash hands after use, make essence by indirect method), Morion Quartz, Orgonite, Rutilated Quartz, Shieldite, Smoky Elestial Quartz, Smoky Quartz, Snakeskin Pyrite, Sodalite, Sunshine Aura Quartz, Tourmalinated Quartz, Valentinite and Stibnite. *Chakra:* dantien, earth, spleen. Place in environment.

Toxins: see Detoxification page 188. *Chakra:* earth star, spleen

disperse: Actinolite, Aegerine, Ametrine, Banded Agate, Barite, Blue Quartz, Celestite, Celestobarite, Champagne Aura Quartz, Chinese Chromium Quartz, Chlorite Quartz, Chrysanthemum Stone, Conichalcite, Covellite, Danburite with Chlorite, Eilat Stone, Epidote, Eye of the Storm, Fairy Quartz, Fiskenaesset Ruby, Golden Danburite, Halite, Hanksite, Huebnerite, Iolite, Leopardskin Serpentine, Morion, Ocean Jasper, Orgonite, Pearl Spa Dolomite, Poppy Jasper, Pumice, Pyrite in Quartz, Quantum Quattro, Seraphinite, Serpentine, Shieldite, Smoky Elestial Quartz, Smoky Herkimer, Snakeskin Pyrite, Sodalite, Spirit Quartz, Yellow Apatite. *Chakra:* base, earth star, dantien, spleen, solar plexus

disperse from environment: Chlorite Quartz, Chrysanthemum Stone, Orgonite, Shieldite, Shungite, Sodalite

remove: Ametrine, Celestite, Chlorite Quartz, Iolite, Moss Agate, Orgonite, Serpentine, Shieldite, Sodalite, Shungite, Yellow Apatite. *Chakra:* base, earth, spleen, solar plexus

strengthen resistance to: Beryl, Eye of the Storm, Klinoptilolith (wash hands after use, make essence by indirect method), Ocean Jasper, Pyrite in Quartz, Shungite. *Chakra:* base, earth star, dantien, spleen, solar plexus

---

Unless otherwise directed, place crystal in the environment or on a map, apply over an organ or site of symptom, place on an appropriate chakra, wear as jewellery, or bathe with or use as crystal essence.

Travel support: Orgonite, Preseli Bluestone, Shieldite, Shungite, Smoky Quartz

Tumours: Beta Quartz, Bloodstone, Chlorite Quartz, Klinoptilolith (wash hands after use, make essence by indirect method), Lepidocrosite, Llanoite, Malachite (use as polished stone, make essence by indirect method), Petalite, Quantum Quattro, Quartz with carbon inclusions, Que Sera, Selenite, Seraphinite, Tibetan Quartz

- U -

Ulcers: Ametrine, Blue Siberian Quartz, Calcite, Chrysocolla, Cryolite, Fluorite, Green Aventurine, Hemimorphite, Montebrasite, Moonstone, Peridot, Quantum Quattro, Rhodonite, Sapphire, Siberian Quartz, Tiger's Eye, Tourmaline

    eyes: Sapphire, Tourmaline, Vivianite

    gastric: Agate, Ametrine

    intestinal: Bismuth, Blue Lace Agate, Emerald, Gaspeite, Honey Calcite, Peridot, Rhodonite, Sapphire, Siberian Blue Quartz, Sunstone

    skin: Blue Lace Agate, Calcite, Emerald, Ruby

    stomach: Blue Siberian Quartz

    throat: Chrysocolla

    varicose: Bastnasite, Bloodstone, Blue Lace Agate, Marialite, Prophecy Stone, Ruby, Scapolite

Ungroundedness: Aztee, Basalt, Celestobarite, Chlorite Quartz, Dragon Stone, Empowerite, Flint, Granite, Graphic Smoky Quartz (Zebra Stone), Hematite, Kambaba Jasper, Mohawkite (use as polished stone, make essence by indirect method), Peanut Wood, Polychrome Jasper, Proustite, Serpentine in Obsidian, Shell Jasper, Smoky Elestial Quartz, Steatite, Stromatolite. *Chakra:* earth star, base, dantien. Or place behind knees.

Urinary:

ailments: Amber, Blue Lace Agate, Jadeite, Jasper, Red Calcite, Ruby

system: Citrine, Jade

tract infections: Yellow or Green Zincite according to colour of urine

Unless otherwise directed, place crystal in the environment or on a map, apply over an organ or site of symptom, place on an appropriate chakra, wear as jewellery, or bathe with or use as crystal essence.

- V -

Viral infections: Cathedral Quartz, Himalayan Red Azeztulite, Proustite, Quantum Quattro, Rainforest Jasper, Shaman Quartz, Shungite and see Antiviral page 155. *Chakra:* higher heart

- W -

Wasting diseases: Carnelian, Magnetite (Lodestone), Red Jasper

Water retention: Andean Blue Opal, Bustamite, Halite, Hanksite, Moonstone and see Fluid page 199. *Chakra:* dantien

Weak:

> **energy field:** Celestobarite, Chlorite Quartz, Chrome Diopside, Orgonite, Poppy Jasper, Quantum Quattro, Que Sera, Sedona Stone. Hold between sacral and solar plexus.

> **muscles:** Blue Moonstone and see Muscles page 223

Weather sensitivity: Apricot Quartz, Avalonite, Chlorite Quartz, Golden Healer Quartz, Golden Pietersite, Khutnohorite, Poppy Jasper, Quantum Quattro, Que Sera, Shell Jasper, Shungite, Sillimanite, Silver Leaf Jasper, Strummer Jasper, Wonder Stone. *Chakra:* third eye

Weight:

> **control:** Angelite, Apatite

Unless otherwise directed, place crystal in the environment or on a map, apply over an organ or site of symptom, place on an appropriate chakra, wear as jewellery, or bathe with or use as crystal essence.

loss: Green Tourmaline, Prehnite, Seraphinite, Unakite

over: Kyanite, Green Tourmaline, Seraphinite

under: Danburite

Well-being, promote: Beryllonite, Fiskenaesset Ruby, Fulgarite, Ice Quartz, Keyiapo, Quantum Quattro, Que Sera, Shift Crystal, Strawberry Quartz, Tugtupite, Ussingite. *Chakra:* higher heart

Wound healing: Amber, Cathedral Quartz, Eye of the Storm, Feather Pyrite, Garnet, Quantum Quattro, Que Sera, Schalenblende, Shungite

- X -

X-rays, prevent damage from: Amazonite, Black Moonstone, Chlorite Quartz, Herkimer Diamond, Lepidolite, Malachite (use as polished stone, make essence by indirect method), Malacholla, Orgonite, Shieldite, Shungite, Smoky Elestial Quartz, Smoky Quartz, Smoky Herkimer, Sodalite, Torbernite (use under supervision) and see Radiation page 235. Wear constantly, rub crystal essence over site, take crystal essence frequently.

- Y -

Yin–yang imbalances: Alunite, Celestite, Dalmatian Stone, Day and Night Quartz, Eilat Stone, Hematite with Rutile, Kyanite, Merlinite, Onyx, Poppy Jasper, Morion

---

Unless otherwise directed, place crystal in the environment or on a map, apply over an organ or site of symptom, place on an appropriate chakra, wear as jewellery, or bathe with or use as crystal essence.

Quartz, Scheelite, Shiva Lingam. *Chakra:* base, dantien

- Z -

Zest for life: Bushman Red Cascade, Carnelian, Orange River Quartz, Poppy Jasper, Zebra Stone. *Chakra:* dantien

Zinc absorption: Galena (wash hands after use, make remedy by indirect method). Pyrite in Sphalerite. *Chakra:* solar plexus

Unless otherwise directed, place crystal in the environment or on a map, apply over an organ or site of symptom, place on an appropriate chakra, wear as jewellery, or bathe with or use as crystal essence.

Appendix

Conclusions/precis: "Bioinitiative 2012: A Rationale for Biologically-based Exposure Standards for Low-Intensity Electromagnetic Radiation"

"Overall, these 1800 or so new studies report abnormal gene transcription; genotoxicity and single-and double-strand DNA damage; stress proteins because of the fractal RF-antenna like nature of DNA; chromatin condensation and loss of DNA repair capacity in human stem cells; reduction in free-radical scavengers – particularly melatonin; neurotoxicity in humans and animals, carcinogenicity in humans; serious impacts on human and animal sperm morphology and function; adverse effects on offspring behavior; and effects on brain and cranial bone development in the offspring of animals that are exposed to cell phone radiation during pregnancy. This is only a snapshot of the evidence presented in the BioInitiative 2012 updated report." Research summaries: http://www.bioinitiative.org/report/wp-content/uploads /pdfs/RFR-11_28-research-summary.pdf

The Draper Report: Childhood leukemia study: http://www.emfs.info/The+Science/abstracts/Draper/#2 008, reported and commented on in:

British Medical Journal (2005) Jun 4;330(7503):1290
"Childhood cancer in relation to distance from high voltage power lines in England and Wales: a case-control study."

G. Draper, T. Vincent, MF Kroll, J. Swanson

Conclusions: There is an association between childhood leukaemia and proximity of home address at birth to high voltage power lines, and the apparent risk extends to a greater distance than would have been expected from previous studies. About 4% of children in England and Wales live within 600 m of high voltage lines at birth. If the association is causal, about 1% of childhood leukaemia in England and Wales would be attributable to these lines, though this estimate has considerable statistical uncertainty. There is no accepted biological mechanism to explain the epidemiological results; indeed, the relation may be due to chance or confounding.

British Journal of Cancer (2010) 103, 1122–1127
"Childhood cancer and magnetic fields from high-voltage power lines in England and Wales: a case-control study"

ME Kroll, J. Swanson, TJ Vincent and GJ Draper, University of Oxford, Childhood Cancer Research

Group, Richards Building, Old Road Campus, Headington, Oxford OX3 7LG, UK; 2 National Grid, 1–3 Strand, London WC2N

Conclusion: Although not statistically significant, the estimate for childhood leukaemia resembles results of comparable studies. Assuming causality, the estimated attributable risk is below one case per year. Magnetic-field exposure during the year of birth is unlikely to be the whole cause of the association with distance from overhead power lines previously reported from this study.

British Journal of Cancer (2012) Sep 11. doi: 10.1038/bjc.2012.359. [Epub ahead of print]
"Case-control study of paternal occupation and childhood leukaemia in Great Britain, 1962–2006."

TJ Keegan, KJ Bunch, TJ Vincent, JC King, KA O'Neill, GM Kendall, A. MacCarthy, NT Fear, MF Murphy

Conclusion: Our results showed some support for a positive association between childhood leukaemia risk and paternal occupation involving social contact. Additionally, LL risk increased with higher paternal occupational social class.

References

1. See Henshaw: http://www.electric-fields.bris.ac.uk/ (consulted April 2014)

2. The Computer Clear program was designed by World Development System. Further details can be found at www.computerclear.com

3. Dulwich Health: http://www.rolfgordon.co.uk/ (consulted April 2014)

4. See the Research section and Appendix.

5. T. Saunders, Health hazards and electromagnetic fields: http://www.sciencedirect.com/science/article/pii/S1353611703000866
and see Appendix and http://www.karger.com/Article/Abstract/88624 "Biomedical Evidence of Influence of Geopathic Zones on the Human Body: Scientifically Traceable Effects and Ways of Harmonization" (consulted April 2014)

6. Electrosensitivity UK: http://www.es-uk.info/about/denis.html
and http://www.whale.to/a/henshaw.html (consulted April 2014)

7. See Bird, Christopher, *The Divining Hand: The 500 Year-Old Mystery of Dowsing* (1979, Schiffer

Publishing, Revised 1994).

8. See Newman, Hugh, *Earth Grids: The Secret Pattern of Gaia's Sacred Sites* (Wooden Books).

9. *Indian Journal of Research* (2011)5,49–53, Anvikshiki Issn 0973–9777, Advance Access publication, 23 Aug 2011 (see Research Findings Reports for full reference). Consulted April 2014.

10. See Appendix and Research

11. See research summaries: http://www.bioinitiative .org/report/wp-content/uploads/pdfs/RFR-11_28-research-summary.pdf (consulted April 2014)

12. "The Sensitivity of Children to Electromagnetic Fields", Leeka Kheifets, Michael Repacholi, Rick Saunders, Emilie van Deventer: http://pediatrics.aap publications.org/content/116/2/e303.short

13. "Microscope system and screening method for drugs, physical therapies and biohazards", Erlend Hodneland, Hans-Hermann Gerdes, US 20090081775 A1, March 26 2009: http://www.google.com/patents /US20090081775 (consulted April 2014)

14. My thanks to Nicky Crocker for sharing this information and giving permission for its use in this book: http://www.clearenergyhomes.com/symptoms/the-6-stages/

15. "Nurturing Life in Classical Chinese Medicine: Sun Simiao on Healing without Drugs, Transforming Bodies and Cultivating Life", translated by Sabine Wilms, *Journal of Chinese Medicine*, consulted April 2014: http://www.jcm.co.uk/samplearticles/product

/catalog/product/view/10293/nurturing-life-in-classical-chinese-medicine-sun-simiao-on-healing-without-drugs-transforming-bodies-and-cultivating-life/

16. See Lucas, Winafred Blake, *Regression Therapy: A Handbook for Professionals* (Deep Forest Press, Crest Park CA 1993), Vol. 1 p. 65ff

17. See for instance the work of Dr Valerie Hunt and her book *Infinite Mind* (no longer in print but available as an e-book from her website): http://www.valerie vhunt.com/ValerieVHunt.com/Valerie_Hunt_EdD.ht ml (consulted April 2014)

18. http://www.earthspectrum.com/healing/scalar-energy-system.htm (consulted April 2014)

19. See Martino, Regina, *Shungite, Protection, Healing and Detoxification* translated by Jack Cain (Healing Arts Press, Rochester, Vermont 2011) for this and other research and also http://www.earth-products.co.uk /shungite-product

Resources

Crystals:

High vibration crystals, earth healers and other crystals specially charged up for you by Judy Hall are available from www.angeladditions.co.uk

Trigonics, Eye of the Storm (Judy's Jasper) and just about everything else can be obtained from John van Rees: www.exquisitecrystals.com

Shungite products are available from www.earth-products.co.uk and www.angeladditions.co.uk

Orgonite is available from www.Lilpictureplace.com, http://www.ebay.co.uk/usr/anturioart, and www.ksc.crystals.

Essences:

Petaltone crystal cleansing and recharging essences: www.petaltone.co.uk

Crystal Balance cleansing and recharging essences: www.crystalbalance.net

Green Man Tree Essences, Shungite and Shield 1:
www.greenmantrees.demon.co.uk

Relevant books by Judy Hall and other authors:

By Judy Hall
*Earth Blessings: Using Crystals for Personal Energy Clearing,
Earth Healing and Environmental Enhancement*
Crystal Bible vols 1–3
The Crystal Wisdom Oracle
Crystals and Sacred Sites
Life Changing Crystals
101 Power Crystals
The Crystal Experience
Crystal Practicalities, DVD: www.angeladditions.co.uk

By Others
Gordon, Rolf *Are You Sleeping in a Safe Place?* Dulwich
Health Society, 1988. ISBN 09514017 0 X

Martino, Regina *Shungite, Protection, Healing and
Detoxification* translated by Jack Cain, Healing Arts Press,
Rochester, Vermont 2011

Newman, Hugh *Earth Grids: The Secret Patterns of Gaia's
Sacred Sites*, Wooden Books

Anti-geopathic devices and practitioners

Nicky Crocker, New Zealand:
http://www.clearenergyhomes.com/
Rolf Gordon, anti-geopathic stress products:
http://www.dulwichhealth.com/
Computer Clear programme:
www.computerclear.com
Bailey Geopathic Stressbuster:
http://www.baileyessences.com/geopathic-stress/geo
pathic-stressbuster/

Articles/websites

Earth Currents – as Pathogenic Agents for Illness and the Development of Cancer, Freiherr Gustav von Pohl, Freich Verlag, Feucht, 1983 (out of print)

Dr Valerie Hunt, *Infinite Mind* (out of print but available via website): http://www.valerievhunt.com/ValerieVHun t.com/Valerie_Hunt_EdD.html

http://www.dailymail.co.uk/femail/article-2331369/The-women-say-allergic-modern-life-Blinding-headaches-Violent-sickness-Even-blackouts-So-wi-fi-mobile-phones-TV-screens-blame.html?ito=feeds-newsxml

"Zeolite: Powerful New Supplement from Volcanic Rock", New Horizons, Brewer Science Library, http://www.mwt.net/~drbrewer/zeolite.htm Includes research sources.

"What is cellular zeolite?" http://www.cancerresearch
uk.org/cancer-help/about-cancer/cancer-questions/what-
is-cellular-zeolite

"Cancer killers": http://www.cancerfightingstrategies
.com/cancer-killers.html#sthash.K51fpsm9.dpbs

Nova, Science in the News, Australian Academy of
Science, "The many potential uses of fullerenes: chemical
sponges": http://www.sciencearchive.org.au/nova/024/
024box02.html

Research Findings Reports

Consulted April 2014 unless otherwise specified.

Useful bibliography: "Guidelines for Earth Energy Analysis" by Alex Stark.
http://alexstark.com/guidelines/earth-energy

Study by Bristol University, Professor Denis L. Henshaw: http://www.electric-fields.bris.ac.uk/ http://powerwatch .org.uk/columns/henshaw/index.asp and http://www.powerwatch.org.uk/elf/overview.asp

For an explanation by Henshaw of how the effects operate: http://www.whale.to/a/henshaw.html
http://www.electrosensitivity.org.uk/
http://powerwatch.org.uk/rf/phones.asp

Matthews, JC, Buckley, AJ, Wright, MD and Henshaw, DL, 2012, "Comparisons of ground level measurements of ion concentration and potential gradient upwind and downwind of HV power lines in corona". *Journal of Electrostatics*, vol 70, pp. 407–417

Matthews, JC, Ward, JP, Keitch, PA and Henshaw, DL, 2010, "Corona ion induced atmospheric potential gradient perturbations near high voltage power lines". *Atmospheric Environment*, vol 44, pp. 5093–5100

Matthews, JC and Henshaw, DL 2009, "Measurements of atmospheric potential gradient fluctuations caused by corona ions near high voltage power lines". *Journal of Electrostatics*, vol 67, pp. 488–491

Matthews, JC, Buckley, AJ, Keitch, PA, Wright, MD and Henshaw, DL 2009, "Measurements of corona ion induced atmospheric electricity modification near to HV power lines" in: N Green (eds) *ELECTROSTATICS 2007*. Deutsche Physikalische Gesellschaft and IOP Publishing Ltd, Bristol

Henshaw, DL, Ward, JP and Matthews, JC, 2008, "Can disturbances in the atmospheric electric field created by powerline corona ions disrupt melatonin production in the pineal gland?" *J Pineal Res*, vol 45, pp. 341–350

Oxford University EMF effects study: http://wwwemfs .info/The+Science/Research/Draper/

Response to Oxford University childhood leukaemia study: http://www.emfs.info/The+Science/Research/Draper/Responses+to+Draper.htm

For a comprehensive list of research findings go to:

EMFields: http://www.emfields.org/faq.asp

Earth Spectrum Health: http://www.earthspectrum.com/healing/scalar-energy-system.htm

Interesting articles and reports of the latest research findings: www.emfblues.com

Tetrawatch: http://www.tetrawatch.net/links/links.php?id=health&list=frequency

"How Exposure to GSM & TETRA Base-station Radiation can Adversely Affect Humans", GJ Hyland, August 2002, Associate Fellow University of Warwick, UK: http://www.psrast.org/mobileng/hylandbasestation.pdf

"iPad and phone dangers for kids | EMFacts Consultancy" www.emfacts.com/2013/12/ipad-and-phone-dangers-for-kids/
18 Dec 2013 – Other relevant links: New Media as Biohazard: http://eunson.net/upload/*biohazard*/ANZCA_2012_Eunson_biohazard.pdf
http://www.emfacts.com/2013/12/ipad-and-phone-dangers-for-kids/

"Secret Report On Cell Phone Dangers And Tetra: Confidential Report On TETRA Strictly For The Police

Federation Of England and Wales" By B. Trower (25.4.2011): http://www.rense.com/general60/tetra.htm

"Health Effects from Radiofrequency Electromagnetic Fields: Report of the independent Advisory Group on Non-ionising Radiation": http://www.hpa.org.uk/webc/hpawebfile/hpaweb_c/1317133827077

"Mobile Phone (Cell Phone) Base Stations and Human Health": http://www.mcw.edu/radiationoncology/ourdepartment/radiationbiology/Mobile-Phone-Cell-Phone-Base-S.htm

"Energy and Climate Change Committee: Written evidence submitted by John Weigel (SMR78)": http://www.publications.parliament.uk/pa/cm201314/cmselect/cmenergy/161/161vw72.htm

"Childhood Cancer in Relation to Indicators of Magnetic Fields from Ground Current Sources," The associations of cancer with conductive plumbing suggest that cancer risk is increased among persons with elevated magnetic field exposure from residential ground currents." (Nancy Wertheimer, David A. Savitz, Ed Leeper, 1994, Wiley InterScience)

Gustav Freiherr von Pohl: *Erdstrahlen als Krankheitserreger – Forschungen auf Neuland* in 1932 , republished in 1978. The new title also has the wording "Erdstrahlen als

Krebsursache und Krankheitserreger", meaning Earth radiation as cause of cancer and other illnesses. The English title is *Earth Currents – Causative Factor of Cancer and Other Diseases* [ISBN 3772494021] – published in Munich in 1932: http://geopathology-za.wikidot.com /gustav-freiherr-von-pohl

"Geopathic Stress Zones and Their Influence on the Human Organism", Gerhard W. Hacker, Annabell Eder, Christoph Augner, Gernot Pauser, IGGMB – Research Institute for Frontier Questions of Medicine and Biotechnology, Landeskrankenhaus ˙ Salzburg – University Clinicum of the Paracelsus Private Medical University, Salzburg Federal Clinics (SALK), Salzburg, Austria: http://www.med-grenzfragen.eu/download/Geo pathy-Gerhard-Hacker-Lithuania08.pdf

Cell phone studies: http://www.ewg.org/cellphoneradi-ation/executivesummary

Cell phone studies: http://scholar.google.co.uk/scholar?hl=en&q=cell+phone+radiation&btnG=&as_sdt=1%2C5
http://stopsmartmeters.org/wp-content/uploads/2012/03/

"Biological Effects and Safety in Magnetic Resonance Imaging: A Review", Valentina Hartwig, Giulio Giovannetti, Nicola Vanello, Massimo Lombardi, Luigi Landini, and Silvana Simi: http://www.ncbi.nlm.nih .gov/pmc/articles/PMC2705217/

http://bronte.celltowerstudy.com/previous-research/belo-horizonte-municipality-minas-gerais-state-brazil/

http://source.southuniversity.edu/health-risks-of-using-mobile-phones-137310.aspx#sthash.FIVcGHDW.dpuf

"Effects of High-Voltage Power on Birds Breeding within the Powerlines' Electromagnetic Fields", Paul F. Doherty, Jr. and Thomas C. Grubb, Jr. http://audubon-omaha.org/bbbox/nabs/pdtg1.htm

"Properties of Extremely Low Frequency Electromagnetic Fields and their Effects on Mouse Testicular Germ Cells", YS Kim, SK Lee, *International Journal of Oral Biology*, 2010 – KoreaMed, Published in: *Defense Science Research Conference and Expo (DSR), 2011*: http://ieeexplore.ieee.org/xpl/login.jsp?tp=&arnumber=6026859&url=http%3A%2F%2Fieeexplore.ieee.org%2Fxpls%2Fabs_all.jsp%3Farnumber%3D6026859 http://www.koreamed.org/SearchBasic.php?RID=0173IJOB/2010.35.4.137&DT=1

Letter No.V-34564, Reg.533/2007–2008 *Indian Journal of Research* (2011) 5,49–53
Anvikshiki Issn 0973–9777, Advance Access publication 23 Aug 2011, "Effect of Radio Frequency Electromagnetic Fields Emitted By Mobile Phone and Cellular Phone Base Station on Human Health" 49–53, HD Khanna and Rajendra Kumar Joshi

Pediatrics (Official Journal of the American Academy of Pediatrics). "The Sensitivity of Children to Electromagnetic Fields", Leeka Kheifets, Michael Repacholi, Rick Saunders, PhD, Emilie van Deventer, PhD: http://pediatrics.aappublications.org/content/116/2/e303.short

California Health Department, "Report on the Possible Health Risks Associated with Power Frequency Electric and Magnetic Fields (EMFs)": http://www.dhs.ca.gov/ehib/emf/RiskEvaluation/riskeval.html

In the interests of balance and to avoid bias: this site presents the consensual, conventional view as it stood in 1999: Federal Communications Commission, Office of Engineering & Technology, "Questions and Answers about Biological Effects and Potential Hazards of Radiofrequency Electromagnetic Fields", *OET Bulletin* 56, August 1999: http://transition.fcc.gov/Bureaus/Engineering_Technology/Documents/bulletins/oet56/oet56e4.pdf

"Health Problems and Disease Patterns", Authors: Muscat, Joshua, Stellman, Steven D. in *94. Education and Training Services*, McCann, Michael, Editor, *Encyclopedia of Occupational Health and Safety*, Jeanne Mager Stellman, Editor-in-Chief. International Labor Organization, Geneva. © 2011: http://www.ilo.org/oshenc/part-xvii/education-and-training-services/item/706-health-problems-and-disease-patterns?tmpl=component

&print=1

Evaluation of water-treated crystals: http://www.my.vi
tajuwel.com/scientific_report.pdf

In 2012, in Italy, mobile phone devices were added to the
list of Class 2B carcinogens responsible for possible
genetic damage, brain dysfunction, brain tumours and
conditions such as sleep disorders and headaches.
Source: http://www.telegraph.co.uk/health/9619514/
Mobile-phones-can-cause-brain-tumours-court-
rules..html

*New Crystal in the Pineal Gland: Characterization and
Potential Role in Electromechano-Transduction*, Baconnier,
Simon; Lang, Sidney B.; De Seze, Rene – and see the
References in the abstract: http://www.ursi.org/
proceedings/procga02/papers/p2236.pdf

BOOKS

SPIRITUALITY

O is a symbol of the world, of oneness and unity; this eye represents knowledge and insight. We publish titles on general spirituality and living a spiritual life. We aim to inform and help you on your own journey in this life.
If you have enjoyed this book, why not tell other readers by posting a review on your preferred book site?

Recent bestsellers from O-Books are:

Heart of Tantric Sex
Diana Richardson
Revealing Eastern secrets of deep love and intimacy to
Western couples.
Paperback: 978-1-90381-637-0 ebook: 978-1-84694-637-0

Crystal Prescriptions
The A-Z guide to over 1,200 symptoms and their healing
crystals
Judy Hall
The first in the popular series of seven books, this
handy little guide is packed as tight as a pill-bottle with
crystal remedies for ailments.
Paperback: 978-1-90504-740-6 ebook: 978-1-84694-629-5

Take Me To Truth
Undoing the Ego
Nouk Sanchez, Tomas Vieira
The best-selling step-by-step book on shedding the Ego,
using the teachings of *A Course In Miracles*.
Paperback: 978-1-84694-050-7 ebook: 978-1-84694-654-7

The 7 Myths about Love...Actually!
The journey from your HEAD to the HEART of your SOUL
Mike George
Smashes all the myths about LOVE.
Paperback: 978-1-84694-288-4 ebook: 978-1-84694-682-0

The Holy Spirit's Interpretation of the New Testament
A Course in Understanding and Acceptance
Regina Dawn Akers
Following on from the strength of *A Course In Miracles*,
NTI teaches us how to experience the love and oneness
of God.
Paperback: 978-1-84694-085-9 ebook: 978-1-78099-083-5

The Message of A Course In Miracles
A translation of the text in plain language
Elizabeth A. Cronkhite
A translation of *A Course in Miracles* into plain, everyday
language for anyone seeking inner peace. The
companion volume, *Practicing A Course In Miracles*,
offers practical lessons and mentoring.
Paperback: 978-1-84694-319-5 ebook: 978-1-84694-642-4

Thinker's Guide to God
Peter Vardy
An introduction to key issues in the philosophy of
religion.
Paperback: 978-1-90381-622-6

Your Simple Path
Find happiness in every step
Ian Tucker
A guide to helping us reconnect with what is really
important in our lives.
Paperback: 978-1-78279-349-6 ebook: 978-1-78279-348-9

365 Days of Wisdom
Daily Messages To Inspire You Through The Year
Dadi Janki
Daily messages which cool the mind, warm the heart
and guide you along your journey.
Paperback: 978-1-84694-863-3 ebook: 978-1-84694-864-0

Body of Wisdom
Women's Spiritual Power and How it Serves
Hilary Hart
Bringing together the dreams and experiences of women
across the world with today's most visionary spiritual
teachers.
Paperback: 978-1-78099-696-7 ebook: 978-1-78099-695-0

Dying to Be Free
From Enforced Secrecy to Near Death to True
Transformation
Hannah Robinson
After an unexpected accident and near-death
experience, Hannah Robinson found herself radically
transforming her life, while a remarkable new insight
altered her relationship with her father a practising
Catholic priest.
Paperback: 978-1-78535-254-6 ebook: 978-1-78535-255-3

The Ecology of the Soul
A Manual of Peace, Power and Personal Growth for Real
People in the Real World
Aidan Walker
Balance your own inner Ecology of the Soul to regain
your natural state of peace, power and wellbeing.
Paperback: 978-1-78279-850-7 ebook: 978-1-78279-849-1

Not I, Not other than I
The Life and Teachings of Russel Williams
Steve Taylor, Russel Williams
The miraculous life and inspiring teachings of one of the
World's greatest living Sages.
Paperback: 978-1-78279-729-6 ebook: 978-1-78279-728-9

On the Other Side of Love
A Woman's Unconventional Journey Towards Wisdom
Muriel Maufroy
When life has lost all meaning, what do you do?
Paperback: 978-1-78535-281-2 ebook: 978-1-78535-282-9

Practicing A Course In Miracles
A Translation of the Workbook in Plain Language and
With Mentoring Notes
Elizabeth A. Cronkhite
The practical second and third volumes of The Plain-
Language *A Course In Miracles*.
Paperback: 978-1-84694-403-1 ebook: 978-1-78099-072-9

Quantum Bliss
The Quantum Mechanics of Happiness, Abundance, and
Health
George S. Mentz
Quantum Bliss is the breakthrough summary of success
and spirituality secrets that customers have been
waiting for.
Paperback: 978-1-78535-203-4 ebook: 978-1-78535-204-1

The Upside Down Mountain
Mags MacKean
A must-read for anyone weary of chasing success and
happiness – one woman's inspirational journey
swapping the uphill slog for the downhill slope.
Paperback: 978-1-78535-171-6 ebook: 978-1-78535-172-3

Your Personal Tuning Fork
The Endocrine System
Deborah Bates
Discover your body's health secret, the endocrine
system, and 'twang' your way to sustainable health!
Paperback: 978-1-84694-503-8 ebook: 978-1-78099-697-4

Readers of ebooks can buy or view any of these bestsellers by clicking on the live link in the title. Most titles are published in paperback and as an ebook. Paperbacks are available in traditional bookshops. Both print and ebook formats are available online.

Find more titles and sign up to our readers' newsletter at http://www.johnhuntpublishing.com/mind-body-spirit

Follow us on Facebook at https://www.facebook.com/OBooks/